THE *ULTIMATE* GUIDE TO PARKRUN

THE ULTIMATE GUIDE TO PARKRUN

Everything You Need to Know About the Friendliest 5K in the World

LUCY WATERLOW

Canbury

First published by Canbury Press 2024
Canbury Press
Kingston upon Thames,
Surrey, United Kingdom

Cover design: Jet Purdie. Cover photo: Graham Smith.

Typesetting: Megan Sheer

Printed and bound in Malta by Gutenberg Press

Where not otherwise stated, photographs have been
provided by parkrun HQ and/or participants

This is a work of non-fiction.

ISBN: 9781914487361

www.canburypress.com
Telling the real story since 2013

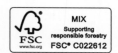

CONTENTS

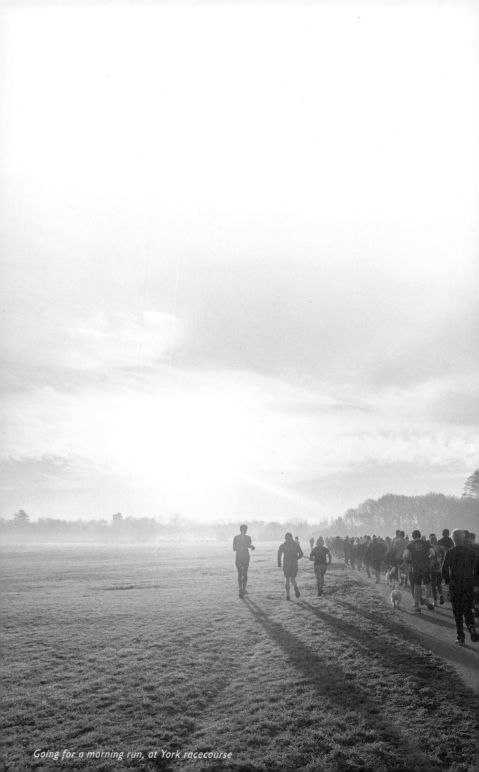

Going for a morning run, at York racecourse

INTRODUCTION

Once upon a time, eight men and five women took part in a 5k time trial organised by a friend in a local park. Little did they know that they had set in motion a worldwide health phenomenon which would go on to span five continents and benefit millions of people. Now every week on Saturday mornings around the globe, hundreds of thousands of people gather for a 3.1 mile timed event, supported by enthusiastic volunteers. It's free to take part in and open to all backgrounds and abilities. This is parkrun (always with a lower case 'p') and it has changed many people's lives for the better.

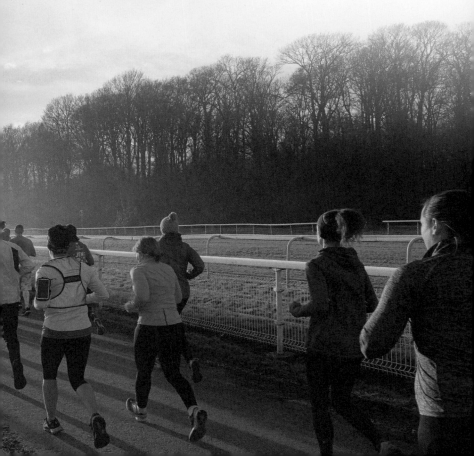

Despite the name, parkrun doesn't have to be a run. And you don't have to be fast. The average finishing time in the UK is 29 minutes 18 seconds. You can walk the whole way if you like. You can join in every week or just occasionally. You can take part with your dog, with your children, with a buggy or a wheelchair, or with a guide runner. You can join in on Christmas Day, in fancy dress, or while on holiday. You can try and finish as fast as you can, or run as many different events as you can. You can even run backwards all the way if you like (yes, there is a parkrunner who does this regularly!).

For some parkrun is just a run, for others it is a way of life, a means of feeling connected to their local community, and an opportunity to spend time with friends and family in the great outdoors. If you're reading this you may already have taken part in at least one parkrun – or intend to. So, if you are looking for some advice on how to lower your time or raise your age grading, get some inspiration to walk, run or volunteer, or find out how you can complete a parkrun challenge – or simply want to know about parkrun's extraordinary story – you are in the right place. This unofficial guide to parkrun is all about celebrating the 'feel-good movement' and the people who have made parkrun what it is today. Enjoy reading and when you put the book down to go for a parkrun, DFYB (Don't Forget Your Barcode!)

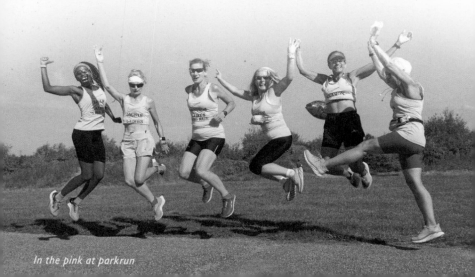

In the pink at parkrun

PARKRUN JARGON BUSTER

Here are some common phrases you will come across in the Guide, and at a parkrun, and what they mean...

A-Z/Alphabet challenge: Completing a parkrun that begins with every letter of the alphabet, eg taking part in Bushy parkrun would tick off a 'B'

Event: Every parkrun held each week is known as an 'event'

First Timer: Someone who takes part in a parkrun for the first time ever, or the first time at a new venue

Home parkrun: The closest parkrun to where you live

junior parkrun: Separate events 2k in distance held on Sunday mornings for 4-14-year-olds

Milestones: A target number of parkruns to work towards to gain official parkrun reward merchandise

parkrun Tourist: Someone who attends a parkrun that isn't their home event

parkwalker: A volunteer who walks the course but doesn't need to be at the very back of the field

PB: Personal Best, the fastest time you have run for a parkrun

RD: Race Director. A volunteer in overall charge of each parkrun event

Tail Walker: A volunteer who walks at the back of the field so nobody ever finishes last

Volunteers: People who undertake unpaid roles to ensure the smooth-running of a parkrun event eg by marshalling

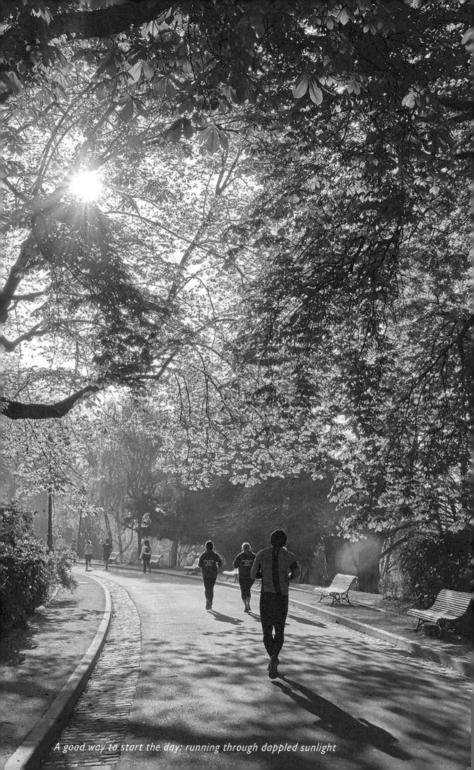

A good way to start the day: running through dappled sunlight

CHAPTER ONE

HOW IT STARTED...
AND HOW IT IS GOING

SMALL BEGINNINGS

The very first event on Saturday, 2 October, 2004 in London's Bushy Park wasn't that much different to how the events are staged today, albeit on a much smaller scale and with less equipment. It was organised by a talented marathoner, Paul Sinton-Hewitt, when he was aged 44 and at a very low point in his life. Or as he once put it: 'My life was in the toilet.' He had been fired from his job as the marketing director of a software company, was divorced, and had picked up an injury which meant he couldn't run. He found this particularly difficult as running had always been a big part of his life. He had grown up doing the sport in South Africa where he ran competitively, and then joined Stragglers Running Club and Ranelagh Harriers when he moved to West London in the 90s. So, not only did he miss the physical and mental health benefits he gained from running, he missed the social side of meeting friends for a run and going for a coffee afterwards. So he decided to do something about it. He invited runners from his local clubs to attend a weekly 5-kilometre run he had plotted through Bushy Park, a royal deer park in the South-West London suburbs. 'This weekly event is for all runners of every discipline who want to measure their performance improvements over a period of

time. A fun event open to all runners,' the original invitation declared. Thirteen runners took part in the inaugural 'Bushy Park Time Trial' (as it was called then). Paul's now wife, Joanne, and three others agreed to help him out to ensure the smooth running of the event, a precursor to how important willing volunteers would become to parkrun's success.

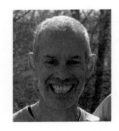

Founder Paul Sinton-Hewitt

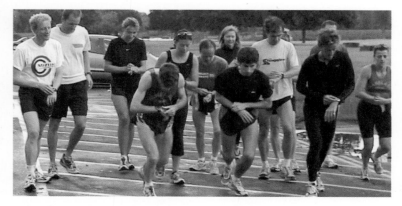

parkrun Pioneers: The very first parkrun in 2004, in Bushy Park, west London

Paul timed the runners, then at the finish, he gave each participant a token with their position. Paul had sourced these from a local hardware store and bashed the finishing numbers on to them using a stamp. The runners then had to handwrite their name and finishing position on a piece of paper on a clipboard in the boot of Paul's car. They left their email addresses so he could send them the full results later.

As the original invitation stated, Paul never intended for this to be a one-off event. His grand plan was to repeat it every Saturday morning, whatever the weather, as a means for runners to unite and track their progress over the distance. It wasn't a race, but a 'timed fun run in a pleasant surrounding'. He was so committed to keeping it going, he didn't go on holiday for three years. As he was unemployed at the time, it gave him a purpose and a focus and a way to 'give something back' to the running community. Word spread – slowly at first – so for the first year the time trial still only averaged about 30 participants each week, some were elite athletes such as Olympic medallist Sonia O'Sullivan. The number of participants steadily increased so by the second anniversary 378 took part. After that, the average attendance continued to be in the hundreds each week. Paul's persistence had paid off but now the numbers were becoming harder to manage. So in January 2007, it was suggested a second event should be set up in another large park nearby, Wimbledon Common. Jim Desmond, another Straggler and a friend of Paul's, took the reins on this one. Part of the idea of this was to help alleviate the large numbers now flocking to Bushy for the time trial. Wimbledon was another resounding success, and when Paul and the inaugural runners realised that this was something that could grow and grow. When others in the running community around England heard about it, they sought Paul's advice on how they could set up similar time trials in their areas. By the end of 2007 there were seven events. A year later this number doubled and the following year

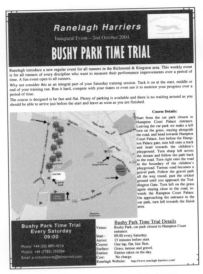

The flyer for that first 'time trial' in 2004

it doubled again. The events just kept growing and growing, attracting the support and sponsorship of major sports companies and individuals, and expanding into all parts of the UK with events in Scotland, Wales, Northern Ireland, and even in the Falkland Islands, a British territory in the South Atlantic.

FROM TIME TRIAL TO PARKRUN

In 2008, the 'time trial' was rebranded as 'parkrun' to make the events sound less competitive and more accessible. It worked. While the time trials had tended to attract people who already identified themselves as runners or were members of athletics clubs, the new parkrun format began to attract people who previously never considered themselves sporty. The culture of inclusivity and the fact it was free spurred

DID YOU KNOW?
Before he became a global running superstar, Mo Farah was the first finisher at the Bushy Park Time Trial on 19th November 2005, with a time of 15.06, out of a field of 66.

DID YOU KNOW?

To the chagrin of grammatical purists, the 'p' of parkrun is lowercase in their branding despite it being a title, and it is always one word, not two.

people who might not normally be able to exercise with others into taking part. The inclusivity didn't just extend to participants, but to venues too. So a parkrun didn't – and doesn't – actually have to be run in a park. Some parkruns are in forests, others around lakes and reservoirs, many are on beaches, and a few on mountains and even volcanoes. Some are held within the grounds of stately homes, in nature reserves, golf courses and in vineyards. In 2017, the first parkrun was launched in a prison in Cumbria, and more prison parkruns have since followed (these are closed events not open to the public). In 2008, parkrun went global and non-UK parkruns started springing up around the world spreading to Africa, Australia and America. parkrun now operates in 21 countries (and counting) spanning five continents.

Two decades on from that first Time Trial, attendance figures have rocketed along with the number of locations. There are more than 2,200 events, with more than 250,000 people taking part every week. By 2023, there had been over nine million registrations, six million unique participants and 800,000 different people volunteering worldwide. Back at Bushy Park where it all started with just 13 runners, 1,381 people finish each week on average, with the highest attendance (yet) in 2019 of 2,545.

'WE WERE THERE FROM THE START!'

Could Paul and his running friends ever have imagined how big the Time Trial would become? Andrew Lane, 67, a retired accountant who now lives in Norfolk, was one of the 13 runners who took part in the very first event.

He recalled: 'I used to live in Teddington, a mile from Bushy Park, and Paul and I became good friends after we met at the Stragglers

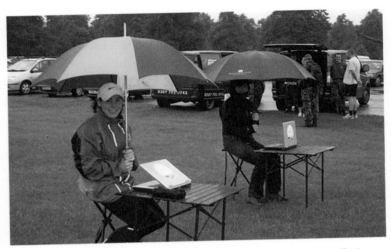

Volunteers using laptops to log finishers in the early days of the Bushy Park Time Trial

Running Club. We used to run together regularly and he often told me how he'd love to set up a Time Trial as these had been popular in South Africa where he grew up. He missed doing them, and then when he became injured, he missed his running friends. His time out on the injury bench gave him the time to finally organise it. He spent several months planning and had originally intended to do it in London's Richmond Park. So he did a lot of reconnaissance for a route there. I can't remember the reason why he changed his mind (later a successful parkrun was set up there) but he settled on Bushy Park for the first one. It was all very unofficial, there was no need to get the permission of the landowner as it was just a group of friends meeting for a run. Another comic bit of the early days is that the start of the route was actually in a car park and we ran across the entrance waving at any drivers coming in to wait for us. That has obviously now changed!'

Andrew revealed: 'I can actually lay claim to helping determine the start time as I remember talking to Paul about it and he said, "I think we'll start at 8am as that's what we did in South Africa". I told him: "Paul, you are starting in English Autumn. People won't come if it is 8am!" A 9am start also felt better than 10am or 11am as then everyone is done and dusted in plenty of time for the rest of their weekend. Some members of Ranelagh Harriers suggested Paul just make it once a month rather than once a week but Paul was adamant it should be weekly. He didn't think it would catch on if it was monthly, as if for example you said it was the first Saturday in the month, people would keep scratching their heads over whether it was the right Saturday to go along, and then it would never get the momentum that it needed. He also had in mind the memory from South Africa where the time trials were weekly. It turned out to be a really good decision.'

Thinking back to that first event which has gone down in parkrun history, Andrew admitted: 'It was all a bit of an anti-climax. I was chairman of the Stragglers Running Club at the time and had done quite a lot of publicity to promote it. But then on the day, only 13 of us turned up which I thought was a bit pathetic. I thought, "poor Paul, he has been telling us about this for months".'

Mike Tivnen, 69, who lives in Teddington and is another member of Stragglers Running Club, was one of the invitees. But the wet weather on that October morning put him off attending the inaugural event.

'I only live a mile away from the park so I was planning to do it,' he says. 'But I looked out the window that morning and it was raining. I thought: "I can't be bothered to go. It's no big deal, it's just Paul organising a run." It is now one of my biggest regrets in life that I missed the opportunity to be one of the original parkrunners!'

Andrew admits he can't recall that much about the actual run: 'I can't really remember anything specific about it as I ran around that park every week. I do remember running 19.48 and I was in fourth place. There was a big gap of about 30 seconds to the person ahead of me and another gap of 30 seconds to the person behind me, so it was very spread out, not at all like today. The slowest time was just under 30 minutes. Paul timed us, gave out his hand-stamped washers and then we went and wrote our details on the clipboard in his car boot and he emailed us all with the results later.'

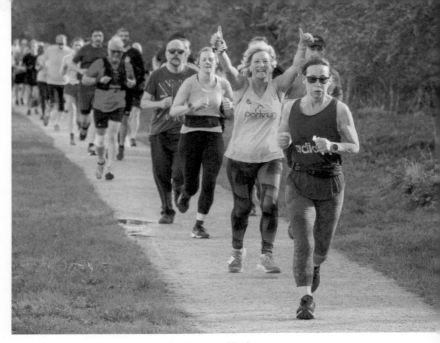

parkrun has gone from a single run in London to worldwide success

Speaking of the low turnout, Andrew said: 'Paul was completely unfazed about it. He just shrugged his shoulders and said "that's fine. I'll keep publicising it and see you next week". I admire him so much for his persistence. The following week 14 people went and the week after that only 11 – the lowest turnout in the event's history. This was before the days of social media so Paul kept advertising it via the running clubs and the email mailing list he was able to create from those who took part and left their addresses. Another clever thing he did in the early days was to write a press release that he sent to the local papers. This definitely helped spread the word. It was so beautifully informal because of Paul's simple but genius idea that allowed people to just turn up without having to register first and get a number to pin on your top like you have to do in most races. Paul registered the runners after they had run by taking down their details and finishing position.'

Mike attended his first time trial in mid November (the eighth event) after some encouragement from his club mates. 'They told

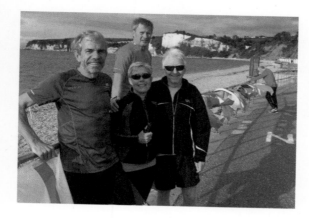

Andrew Lane (left), one of the original parkrunners, and Mike Tivnen (right), who started soon after, with friends after completing a parkrun

me "it's really good, you should come along, we all do the run and go for a coffee afterwards,'" Mike recalled. 'The first time I went, there were 17 finishers. I was 13th in a time of 21.35, which shows that at that time we were all decent runners. None of us had any idea how big it would become. It started off so slowly – mostly 30-50 people in the first year – and then just mushroomed.'

Andrew chuckles. 'I never expected it to become as big as it did. I remember saying to people in the early days, "it is going well but it will never get more than 200 runners as people will find it too crowded and won't want to run on a congested, narrow path". I couldn't have been more wrong! I started noticing how successful it could be when I saw how many families were coming along and running together. That's when I started to think "this appeals to more than just club runners. This is something special".'

Andrew recalls that on the day of the first anniversary more than one hundred took part for the first time. 'Paul had decided to make a big celebration of it – which has continued on anniversaries both of parkrun events and for individual milestones – to today. He got T-shirts and encouraged people to come and bring a picnic. The numbers dropped again after that but not to as low a level as before. Then from 2006 onwards, there were regularly more than a hundred and it just kept growing. In the early days, some running clubs were a bit worried that it would draw people away from club events and stop people doing things like cross country league races on a Saturday. But that never materialised. As we have seen over the years, it actually brings people into running and exercise who go on to join clubs and compete in various races for them. It complements, rather than competes with running club events.'

Mike spent a few years away from the running scene from 2009 while he had surgery on his knees, and when he returned, he was stunned by the transformation in the time trials.

'When I could run again in 2011, I went along one Saturday and it had totally changed. Now it was called parkrun and there were all these people there − kids, people of all sizes, people just joining in with their mates. I thought, "wow, this is amazing!" That was the point I fell in love with it. I stopped thinking of it as "just another run" − although I was still keen to challenge myself and go as fast as I could. I then got my son, Harry, involved and he did his first one with me aged 11 − and he beat me! Years later, he went on to be the first finisher at Bushy a couple of times after getting his PB down to under 16 minutes, and he's run a 2.32 marathon. parkrun is a lot of the reason why he became such a great runner.'

Andrew then witnessed the way the events were managed had to evolve with the increasing numbers, and this was made possible thanks to Paul being so tech-savvy. 'With the numbers increasing, Paul was finding it difficult to register people after running, especially after the Wimbledon event started too and he was then trying to merge his two databases,' he said. 'He had swapped his clipboard for a laptop early on but then started needing more than one laptop. I remember volunteering one week when numbers had reached the hundreds and there were five long queues of people waiting to register their names and finishing times with five of us who had laptops perched on logs. Paul looked around for answers to this and somehow latched onto barcodes which people could sign up for once, and then use for every run. This came to all of us as a brilliant surprise − something like a supermarket barcode could be used for this.'

Mike, who has now done nearly 400 parkruns and volunteered almost 100 times, agrees it was a genius idea. 'Once you had your

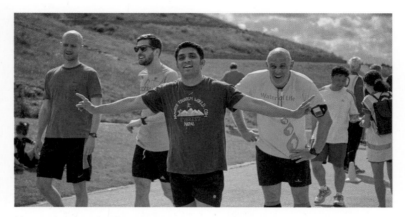

Many parkrunners do different runs wherever they travel at home or abroad

barcode, you knew what to do. You can go whenever you want and then get your results soon after running. I love how it made all the events accessible as it grew too. Nowadays I'll often do a parkrun when travelling to different places in the UK to see friends or on holiday, and I did some in Australia when my son, Ben, lived there'. Speaking of the growth across the UK and overseas, Andrew said Paul started getting requests from people to start time trials where they lived so he would send them the software they needed. 'The events then spread like an infectious disease out of London with people who started setting up their own,' he recalled. There was a real pioneering spirit to parkrun in the early days and it was much more low key than it is now. While he had vital help running the events from his friends including Duncan Gaskell, Jim Desmond, Darren Wood and his now wife, Jo Sinton-Hewitt, Paul Sinton-Hewitt still was orchestrating it all from the shed in his garden and financing it himself. As the events increased, soon the cost of running it outstripped the income, especially when he realised he had to start paying people because some of the work setting up new events was getting too much for anyone to do in their spare time. Andrew said: 'A lot of the early people on the payroll, some of whom have stayed on as paid employees to this day, were the ones who went along and loved parkrun and started helping out just for the love of it. The growth wouldn't have happened without Paul's persistence and tenacity, and it wouldn't have been sustainable without a few other key people who supported it.'

Reflecting on how big parkrun has become, Andrew thinks the distance has been a big factor in its success. 'If it was shorter, a mile long, people might have thought it is not worth turning up for regularly, and if it was longer, it could have put off those who aren't that fit. Volunteering is easy too which makes it accessible to more people,' he said. 'Then the friendship and community part is special. You see this every Saturday: real genuine friendships among the volunteers and participants.'

Having quick results has also helped the event. When Andrew and Mike were road racing 30 years ago, they'd often only get their results a fortnight later by leaving a stamped self addressed envelope on the day. At a parkrun, you usually get your time by midday on the day. Social media played a big part in the growth too, particularly Facebook, which made it easier to spread the word about events and recruit volunteers.

Andrew, who along with others set up Eaton junior parkrun in Norwich in 2015, says this has been another huge success and an excellent way to get children active. 'Through junior parkrun, we are seeing children growing up as parkrunners. There are a couple I used to see as little boys every week in Norwich who have gone on as adults to run 2.30 marathons and 33 minute 10ks. Their achievements wouldn't have happened if they hadn't had the fun and regularity of parkrun every Saturday.'

Andrew now has 530 parkruns and nearly 200 volunteer credits to his name and is thrilled with the 20th anniversary. Previously, all 13 of the 'parkrun pioneers' were reunited at the 10th anniversary celebrations, where they were presented with gold personal barcodes.

DID YOU KNOW?

Paul Sinton-Hewitt was awarded a CBE 'for services to Grassroots Sport Participation' in 2014 and he's now the Executive Director of parkrun.

And where do they think parkrun will be in another 20 years time?

'I think it will keep growing,' Andrew enthuses. 'There are more countries around the world where there is an appetite for it and there are no signs of people getting tired of it. It has become a national treasure.'

THE ALL IMPORTANT BARCODE

Whilst parkrun has tried to move away from the time trial element so people don't feel they have to run fast to attend, the runs are all still timed and the results recorded and published. Gone are the days of pen and paper to keep track. Now all participants are encouraged to register on the parkrun website for an account before taking part. They are then assigned their own personal barcode. This can be printed out, saved on a mobile phone, or you can pay to have it printed on a wristband or shoe tag. You only have to register once, and then you have a free ticket to turn up at any parkrun in the world whenever you like.

Experienced parkrunners will be familiar with the acronym DFYB (Don't Forget Your Barcode) as no barcode means no result – and there are 'no exceptions' to this rule. Anyone taking part who doesn't have a personal barcode scanned will appear in the results as an 'unknown runner'. Their position will be shown but with no further details and no time. This allows people to still take part prior to officially registering (although this isn't encouraged), or if they don't want that particular run to be added to their personal parkrun stats.

However, the barcode is more than just a means of recording times and achievements so every participant is also urged to carry one as a means of keeping safe. If someone gets into trouble when taking part and needs medical assistance, their barcode will enable the emergency services to know who they are and their next of kin via a contact number added to their account when registering.

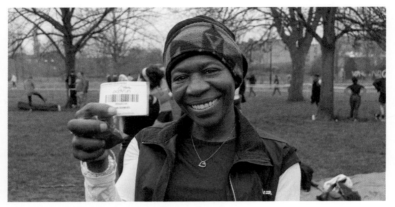

You definitely need your barcode, downloadable for free

Just like in the early days, tokens are handed out with finishing positions but these are now small cards with parkrun branding and another barcode on. Finishers take their token to be scanned by a volunteer at the end of the finishing funnel, and then have their personal barcode scanned. All tokens must be returned so they can be used again the following week. Like magic just a short time later, the participant will receive an email with their finishing time and position in the event, and a link to view the full set of results online.

Thanks to the data collected via barcodes, participants can keep track of every parkrun they have ever run and the progress they have made, including their best and average finishing times and positions.

THE RESULTS DECODED

On the 'latest results' page of every parkrun you can find the full set of finishers for the most recently held event, in finishing order. In the 'compact' view, names, finishing positions and times are all listed, along with the participants' gender and age category. The age groups tend to be shown in four year bands, 30-34, 35-39 etc. If the finisher is a member of a recognised running club, that will be listed here too. If the time was a PB (Personal Best, ie, the fastest they have ever run) for the runner on that particular course, a 'new PB' tag will be shown in red. If it is the runner's debut at that particular parkrun, then a green leaf will be added which represents 'first timer'. By clicking into the 'detailed' results view, you can see more information on each runner. This includes how many parkruns they have ever run, whether they are in a 'milestone club', what gender position they finished, and what their PB is for that course (if their most recent run wasn't their best ever). The 'age grading' is also shown here – and in the results email sent to finishers – as a percentage.

WHAT IS AGE GRADING?

It is a score comparing your time to those of your age and gender worldwide. Each year statisticians at World Masters Athletics use a formula based on global running records to find out the best possible time an athlete can run according to their gender and age. The formula is then used to calculate the percentage, with the higher the score, the better the performance. So to have an age grading of 100 percent or above, you would be the world record holder for your age and gender. At 100 percent, you could also be – or be extremely

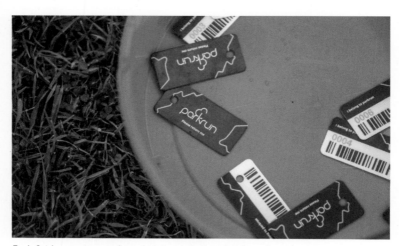

Each finisher receives a token which is matched to their barcode

close to – world record level. A percentage above 90 denotes 'world class level', above 80 percent 'national class level', and 70 percent 'regional class level'. Above 60 percent is 'local class level'. Having age grading means you can level the playing field against others of different genders and generations. So a 40-year-old woman may finish behind a 20-year-old man in a parkrun

with a slower time, but her age grading might be higher, showing she performed better than him relative to their gender and age. Every parkrun venue used to display age graded records on its website, showing the best age graded runs in the event's history to whet the appetite of those who want to be competitive about this, or be amazed/inspired by other people's scores/times. However, they stopped displaying this information at the start of 2024. Participants can still see who had the best age grading in each weekly event though by using a tab on the results to change the display from finishing position to age grading.

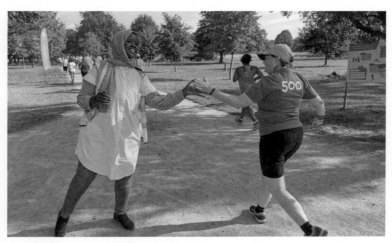

On the way to completing another parkrun

IT'S A RUN, NOT A RACE, OR IS IT?

After setting up the first event as a time trial and not a race, Paul has always been keen to emphasise that parkrun is not a serious competition. Each event has a 'first finisher' but not a 'winner.' And at the other end of the field, there is no last place and no cut-off time. A volunteer Tail Walker always stays at the back of the pack and is recorded in the results so no-one ever has to worry about coming last, or being left behind.

Even though it has never been a race, numerous stats used to appear on every parkrun event page showing the best performances. This included the 'fastest 500' (the top 500 fastest times ever recorded on the course), a list of all the women who had ever run a sub-20 minute time and men who had run a sub-17 minute time, and a roll call of 'first finishers', including how many times they had achieved the accolade. The results were also sent to the Power

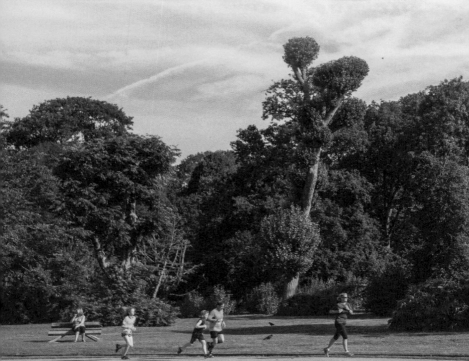

Lovely day for a parkrun. Photo: David Rowe

of 10, a website that records all the races and PBs of British athletes who meet certain performance standards as a means of driving improvement up to world class level.

At the bottom of each parkrun event homepage, you could see at a glance who was the male and female record holder and their finishing time. There also used to be lists on the parkrun UK site showing all the course records across the country, who the first finishers each week were at every event, and who had the best age grading each week across the country.

So for a run that isn't a race, it could actually get quite competitive if you wanted to beat the course record, make the fastest 500 list, or achieve the most first place finishes at that venue. At the start of 2024, parkrun decided to remove all the lists of the fastest 500 runners, first finishers, sub 20/17 minute runners and course and age category records from its websites. You can read more about this decision in Chapter Eight.

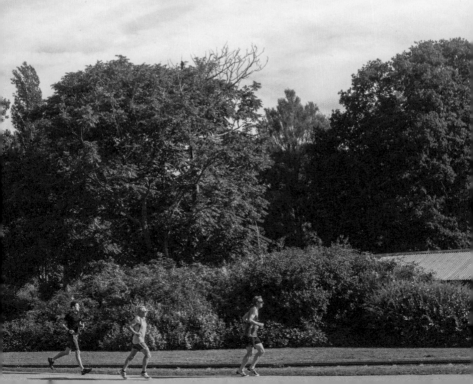

MILESTONE MOMENTS

The 'it's not the winning but the taking part' motto extends to the 'milestones' parkrunners are encouraged to aim for. These reward 'persistence over performance'. Once you have run 25 parkruns you can literally say you have been there, done that and got the T-shirt – as you can buy a parkrun milestone tee. You can then aim to run 50, 100, 250 and 500 to further your T-shirt collection and personal pride in becoming a parkrun stalwart. Many people enjoy celebrating their milestones with their fellow parkrunners by bringing cake to the finish, running in fancy dress or inviting friends and family to run with them.

Volunteers can also start a tally and are celebrated when they reach the milestones of 25, 50 etc times volunteered, with the opportunity to buy celebratory parkrun merchandise too.

Those under the age of 18 reach their first milestone when they have completed 10 parkruns. Marking milestones has proved to be extremely popular to incentivise participation as a runner and volunteer. For many years, milestone T-shirts were given out for free but as parkrun grew and more and more people reached milestones, it became unsustainable and too expensive. In 2021, charging for the T-shirts (at a fixed price of £15 worldwide) was introduced. This opened the doors for a whole shop of milestone merchandising and for parkrun to work with larger retailers to meet the demand for products.

The idea for rewarding attendance was again born where it all started at Bushy. On the second anniversary of what was then still known as the Bushy Park Time Trial, founder Paul Sinton-Hewitt was awarded a black fleece from his fellow runners as a thank you for all he had done to make it possible. He thought it would

DID YOU KNOW?

When stats were kept and celebrated, Andy Baddeley held the world record for the fastest parkrun time of 13:48 for 11 years, until another Andy and fellow Olympian, Andy Butchart, lowered it to 13:45 in 2023.

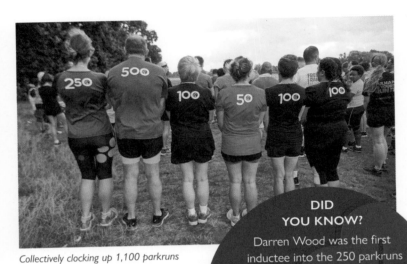

Collectively clocking up 1,100 parkruns

be good to share the love and keep rewarding people for turning up or helping out. He set what he thought was a lofty target of 100 finishes for people to aim for and personally presented the first 20 to reach this milestone with a personalised fleece. It quickly became impossible for him to keep up with the demand and with the help of a sponsor, milestone club jackets were created, and then the T-shirts as we know them today. These were initially handed out by volunteers at the events but again this became unsustainable as events grew in popularity and they are now ordered online and posted.

DID YOU KNOW?

Darren Wood was the first inductee into the 250 parkruns club, reaching the milestone in January 2010. It was then thought it would be such a rare achievement, Paul presented him with a unique top with a gold 250 parkrun logo and a certificate. Now hundreds around the world achieve this milestone every week.

THE PARKRUN WAY

As parkrun rapidly took off and expanded, Paul realised he had to come up with a means of trying to keep it true to his original goals and ensuring the atmosphere at each event was similarly warm and friendly. His vision for parkrun was to create a welcoming community of all abilities, and to make social outdoor activity accessible and enjoyable for everyone. He wrote a 'parkrun code' to share what the ethos of the events should be for those taking part and organising events. This in part is the secret to its success and why 'parkrun tourism' (visiting an event that isn't local to you, perhaps by joining a parkrun near to where you are staying on holiday) is so appealing. You can go somewhere else in the country – or the world – and find the same like-minded people spending their Saturday morning the way you do at home. While all parkruns may have their quirks due to their route or the people who attend, they all follow the same ethos of 'creating an environment that is inclusive, fun and positive,' where you can meet new people and feel part of the local community. Participation covers walking, jogging, running and volunteering and the ethos is that 'each one is equal and all make a contribution to their event'. Whilst inclusivity is a top priority, there are some rules and regulations, which Run Directors might need to enforce or remind people of at events, to ensure the safety of large groups running together. These include, for example, rules over how many dogs a person can run with and what lead they can use (more on this in Chapter Two), not joining in on a bike or scooter, and young children always staying with a parent or guardian. One of parkrun's main principles is to be 'free, for everyone, forever'.

THE PARKRUN CODE FOR PARTICIPANTS AT A GLANCE

- Pay attention to the pre-run briefing
- Under 11s within arm's reach of a parent or guardian
- Respect everyone's right to participate in their own way
- One dog on a short lead per person
- Be mindful of your local environment and other park users
- No barcode, no time, no exception
- Thank the amazing volunteers
- Have fun – it's only a walk, jog or run

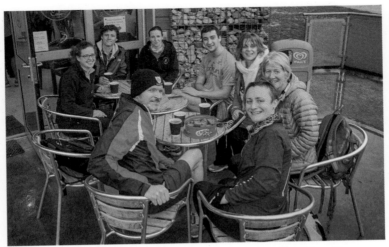

Enjoying a chat and a drink at Northala Fields parkrun in London. Photo: Bruce Li

CAFE CULTURE

When setting up the first time trials, Paul was keen for them to be an opportunity to socialise as well as to exercise. To this end, he encouraged participants to join him afterwards at a nearby cafe for a coffee and catch up. This continued as more time trials, and then parkruns, were established. So while not a prerequisite for a venue, having a place near, or at the location, where parkrunners can go afterwards for food and drink is encouraged. Volunteers often head to the cafe together to process the results and sort out the finishing tokens. Each parkrun event course page lists where the nearest cafes are and invites people to join them there after walking, running or volunteering. For many people the cafe visit afterwards is as much of a Saturday highlight as the parkrun itself.

(NOT) PARKRUN

During the worldwide Covid19 pandemic when lockdowns were in force, parkruns were cancelled around the world for 15 months. During this time, big gatherings had to be avoided to

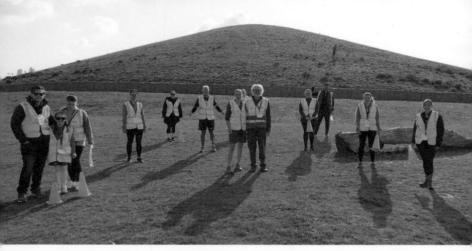

parkrunners are always reminded to thank the volunteers

slow transmission, but getting exercise remained important. To help people still feel connected to their parkrun community and to encourage them to stay active, parkrun introduced '(not)parkrun' – and they are still going. This involves running a 5k wherever and whenever you want, and then adding your time to your parkrun event website. You can do your 5k on the actual parkrun course (which is coined doing a 'freedom' parkrun) or make up your own route. The times are not checked so rely on people being honest with their contributions, which are then displayed in a separate results list on each parkrun event page. These runs are all unofficial and don't count towards parkrun milestones. While (not)parkruns are a lot less popular now actual parkruns are back, the ability to take part in them still remains for those who might not be able to make a Saturday morning event.

NOT EVERYONE'S A FAN

As well as being urged to be kind to one another and respect everyone's right to join in, however they choose, parkrunners are also reminded in the pre-event briefing and 'parkrun code' to be respectful to other park users. Not everyone is delighted to have their space for dog walking, for solitude, or for playing other sports invaded by hundreds of parkrunners every weekend. Equally, residents local to the event locations have to be considered so their streets don't become blocked with parked cars every Saturday morning, and they aren't disturbed by the noise from an event. The environment needs to be considered too, especially as many parkruns are held in areas of outstanding beauty. Volunteers and runners are told to leave the area as they found it with no littering or lost property. Numerous events around the world have been shut down due to the negative impact they have had on a location. In the UK, this was the case with Little Stoke parkrun in Bristol, which was cancelled indefinitely in 2016 after 173 events due to a dispute with the parish council. The council said those taking part must contribute £1 every time they joined in to cover the cost of the 'increased wear' they were causing to the park. In a statement the council said: 'parkrun are an organised group and like any other group using the facilities should contribute towards the maintenance. The parish council has only recently paid out £55,000 from public funds for resurfacing the car park and with the additional 300+ runners per week, will shortly need to replace/repair the path at an estimated cost of £60,000, so as parkrun are significant users of the path on a regular basis they should contribute towards the upkeep.' As a result, parkrun felt it had to close this event as charging those to take part went against its ethos of being free for all.

Heartwood Forest parkrun in Hertfordshire was stopped in 2018 after 47 events. The land it was held on is a developing new forest owned by the Woodland Trust and it was felt it wasn't sustainable for parkrun to continue without adversely affecting this precious area of nature. The Woodland Trust also withdrew its support for Tring parkrun in 2002 after 293 events because Tring Park has sites of Special Scientific Interest and ancient monuments that must be protected. Similarly, in 2017 Hatfield Forest parkrun came to an end after 131 events as the landowners, the National Trust, called for it to be relocated due to parking issues as the event became more and more popular. This is not to imply either the Wood-land Trust or National Trust are unsupportive of parkrun, as other events have been successfully held on their lands for years and many continue to do so. In these instances though, it became clear it wasn't practical as the runs increased in size and could have had lasting damage on the terrain. Other parkruns around the world have come and gone if landowners have withdrawn their consent for them to take place. Having a good relationship with landowners is key for anyone wanting to start a new parkrun.

DOING IT FOR THE KIDS

Children have always been welcome to join in parkruns, with the stipulation that under 11s always be kept within arm's reach of a parent or guardian. But 5k is quite a long way for a young person,

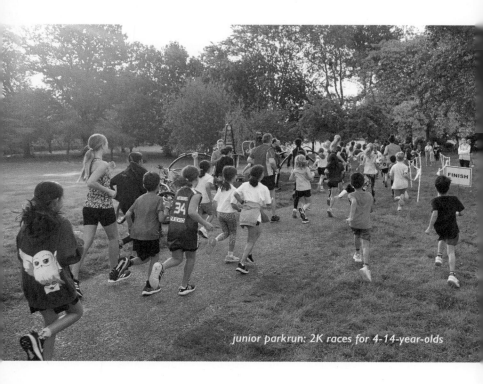

junior parkrun: 2K races for 4-14-year-olds

especially if they want to take part regularly. So in 2010, Paul Graham, an occupational therapist, sports coach and parkrun fan came up with the idea of junior parkrun. These are for 4-14-year-olds and only 2k. Instead of taking place on a Saturday, they are held on a Sunday at 9am. Just like in the grown-up version, the first event was held in Bushy Park with small numbers – just nine children. It soon grew and more were set up around the UK, as well as in Ireland and Australia. Just like the parkruns, the events are timed and finishing position tokens are handed out at the end. Juniors must be registered – for free – for their own barcode to be scanned alongside their finishing token so they can appear in the results. They can work towards milestones of 11 2k runs (the equivalent of a half marathon), 21 (a marathon) and 50 (an ultra-marathon). Children are given a free wristband to commemorate and celebrate their achievement once they reach a milestone, and they can also download a certificate from their account. At junior parkruns, the wristbands are still handed out on the day to make a bigger celebration of a child's achievement, but shy children don't have to go and collect it in front of everyone if they don't want to. Once again, while the run is timed, it isn't designed to be competitive (although try telling some of the speedy youngsters at the front that). The motto is 'it is a run not a race, finish with a smile on your face'. Children are encouraged to run, walk, skip or jump in muddy puddles on their way round, with the aim of enjoying themselves in nature. Young children can be accompanied by their parents or guardians and younger siblings can be pushed around in buggies. Older ones are allowed to run on their own, which they might find preferable if their grown-ups can't keep up with them. No dogs are allowed to join in at junior events and adults aren't allowed to cross the finish line or collect a finish token. Children are encouraged to volunteer too by earning milestones, with many teenagers doing so as part of the Duke of Edinburgh

DID YOU KNOW?

junior parkruns were originally held monthly but now take place every week.

Awards scheme. Giving out high fives as well as lots of cheers is all part of marshalling, with the aim of giving children a positive and happy association with being outside exercising. A difference to the adult parkrun is that all events start with a pre-run warm-up led by a volunteer. This is designed to be a fun way to get children moving and enjoying themselves by doing actions such as star jumps, lunges and windmill arms before they start running/walking.

THE JUNIOR PARKRUN CODE

- A parent or guardian accompanies under 11s to and from the event
- For children aged 4 to 14
- Parents and guardians can take part too
- Please pay attention to the pre-run briefing
- Respect the park and other park users
- Let children walk, jog, skip and run for fun
- No dogs allowed
- Only children to enter the finish funnel
- No barcode, no time, no exception
- Thank the amazing volunteers

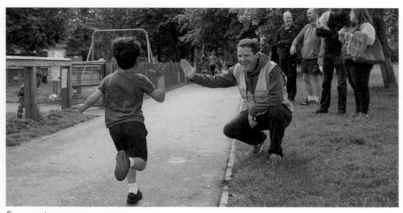

Encouraging younger runners

BRAND PARTNERS

In the early days of parkrun, commercialisation was kept to a minimum and brands who supported it were not given much exposure. But as the organisation grew and more and more parkruns were set up, this approach became unsustainable. While a parkrun is free to take part in, it is not free to put on. Every new parkrun event needs an injection of cash to help get it off the ground, and then there are ongoing running costs, such as for equipment like signs, first aid kits and defibrillators. The development of the parkrun volunteer app cut some event costs. Previously, each event needed stopwatches, expensive barcode scanning machines, and a laptop to download and process the results before they were published. Nowadays, volunteers can just use their own mobile phones for timekeeping, barcode scanning, and results processing, once they've downloaded the free app.

DID YOU KNOW?

It costs the equivalent of £83 per parkrun, per week, to keep events going globally, according to parkrun.

parkrun has big plans to carry on expanding around the world, and to do this it will need more money, which means working with more sponsors and more brand partners. It vets these to ensure they align with its values. Brands are promoted on the organisation's main website, social media channels, and in newsletters to subscribers. Partners over the years have included sports brands, retailers, health and life insurance companies and food and drink makers. parkrun is also supported by a number of official charity partners such as Comic Relief and Mind.

PARKRUN AS A CHARITY

As well as gaining support from other well-established charities, parkrun was registered as a charity in 2018 under the name parkrun Global Ltd. The charity's objectives are listed as 'promoting commu-

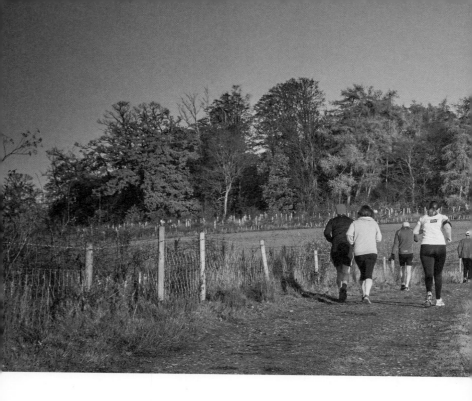

nity participation in healthy recreation by organising and providing running events, creating opportunities for members of the community to participate in and/or volunteer at such running events, and to further such wholly charitable purposes as the trustees may from time to time decide'. In 2023, eight trustees oversaw the work, management and administration of the charity on behalf of its beneficiaries. Charity trustee roles are generally unpaid positions. Data submitted for the end of the 2023 financial year showed that the charity's total income was £7,248,475 and total expenditure £7,302,125.

Just over a third (35.7 per cent) of this income came from their sponsorship deals with its brand partners. It also receives grants, such as from Sport England, and these usually come with rules on how the money can be spent, for example on getting more women or those from low income areas active. parkrun also welcomes donations from individual parkrunners who can give money via any parkrun event page. Individual parkruns can use this to fundraise for specific equip-

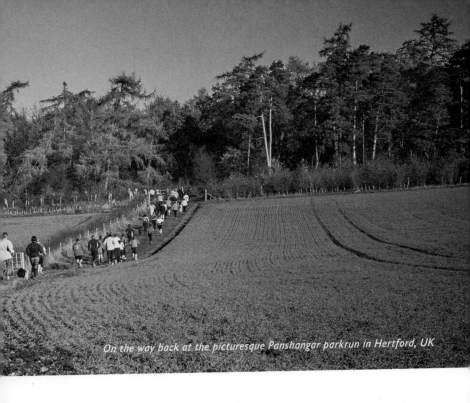

On the way back at the picturesque Panshangar parkrun in Hertford, UK

ment it needs. A big income stream that continues to expand and grow is parkrun's retail offering – charging for parkrun merchandise such as milestone T-shirts and mugs. This made up nearly another third of its income in the year 2022-23 (32.1 percent). This commercial activity is possible due to parkrun setting up a non-charitable subsidiary called parkrun Trading Limited. This company supports parkrun's charitable objectives because all profits are donated to the charity. If you buy any parkrun merchandise, you are supporting the organisation and its events. parkrun is also registered as a limited company, responsible for delivering parkrun in the UK. There are other parkrun registered companies in other countries responsible for delivering parkruns in their areas, such as Australia. In 2024, parkrun had 65 members of paid staff globally, 47 of which are based in the UK, covering roles including management and communications. In the UK, there is a 'senior leadership team' of five people led by Chief Executive Officer, Russ Jefferys. Staff costs accounted for more than a third of expenditure in 2023.

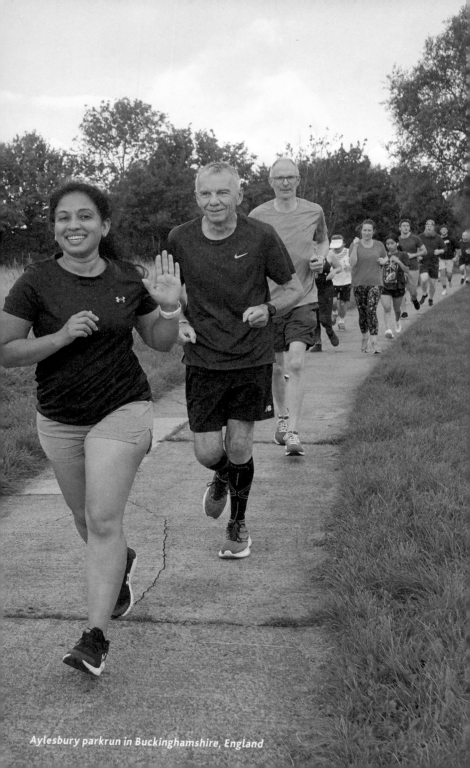

Aylesbury parkrun in Buckinghamshire, England

CHAPTER TWO

MEET THE PARKRUNNERS

parkrun means different things to different people. Some may be running it competitively, others to be sociable. Some are driven by reaching a milestone, others just want to use it as a means to stay fit and healthy. Some take part with their dogs or their children, and others are there to walk rather than run. So here are some of the parkrunners you might meet at your local event, and why they enjoy taking part...

THE FRONT RUNNERS

With its roots as a time trial that published data on the fastest recorded times, some participants treat a parkrun as a race. This might be to test their fitness, to practise running at a target pace for an official race they are training for, or for personal pride in a finishing time, position or age grading. While parkrun no longer publishes statistics on age graded records or lists the fastest 500 parkrunners for each event, participants can still aim to be recorded as the first male or female finisher each week. These records are kept along with the finishing time on the event history page of each parkrun. Finishing as the first female is something that motivates Caroline Wood, a retiree from Hove on England's south coast. Since she first started parkrunning in 2008 when she was in her forties, she has finished first at 114 different events, and she once even finished first overall at Great Salterns parkrun in Portsmouth. 'I love doing different parkruns – the more challenging the better – mud and hills are my thing,' she says. 'I treat a parkrun as a race as it is an opportunity to push myself and compare my time to my peers. Now I'm 60-years-old, first place is

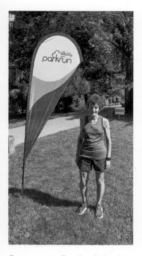

Frontrunner Caroline Wood

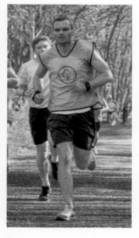

Frontrunner James Mumford

harder to come by but I still aim to finish in the top three, or achieve a high age grading. I hope I inspire other mature female athletes. I also volunteer regularly and love the fact that parkrun is a sociable community. It is whatever you want it to be, whatever your standard.'

James Mumford, 44, a production manager from Huddersfield, West Yorkshire, is another who enjoys the friendly competition parkrun provides. 'I love going to a new parkrun and seeing if I can beat the local regulars. Because of the friendly atmosphere of parkrun, there's always a nice chat afterwards, win or lose,' he says. 'You never know how good the standard will be week to week, so you may get someone winning in 15 minutes, or in over 20 minutes. For someone of my level with a 5k PB of 16.45, this makes it interesting as any week could be winnable. I also find it a great way to try out new shoes and kit for the bigger, more serious, paid races I've entered.'

When he first took up running in his thirties, he was really unfit. 'I was persuaded to try parkrun with my wife's family,' James recalled. 'I didn't like the idea of competing then and I didn't feel like a runner. I felt like an imposter and I was really self conscious. But I got round in 23 minutes and I loved it. parkrun became the gateway for me to really get into running. I kept going back to my local one in Huddersfield and got to sub-18 minutes within a year. I then joined a running club and now it's my passion, my obsession. I'm so grateful that I started running properly at the age 36. I've now done 90 parkruns and finished first in 27 of them.' He said: 'If you'd had told me I would finish first when I first started, I wouldn't have believed you.'

Chris Czora, 40 from Northamptonshire, has run 150 parkruns. He admits he is unlikely to ever finish first as his finishing time is usually around 28 minutes, but he still likes to treat it as a race for his own personal satisfaction. 'I used to race in motocross and karts, so I enjoy that buzz of competition,' he says. 'parkrun is somewhat different as it's a run, not a race, but with it being a timed event it creates a form of competition for me personally, compared to a normal run. As someone who didn't really run in the past, I get satisfaction from placing what for me is a good time, and seeing my finishing positions being far higher than when I started. If I have a bad run, there's always next week.'

For Megan Walker, 29, from Hatfield in Hertfordshire, near London, getting faster at parkruns gave her the confidence to be competitive over other race distances when she took up running following spinal surgery.

'parkrun played a huge part in me getting hooked into running and then racing competitively. I first decided to give running a go in 2015 two years after having an operation to repair my spine using titanium rods following an accident,' she says. Her husband, Barnaby, was already a runner and encouraged her to try parkrun. 'I did my first one – Milton Country parkrun in Cambridge – in 22 minutes,' she says.' I loved the atmosphere and became determined to keep going to improve my time. I enjoyed pushing myself in a not super serious way as I knew it wasn't actually a race. Back then, I was too intimidated to enter the big competitive races. As I got faster and broke 20 minutes, then 19 minutes, it gave me the confidence to enter races on the track and road, and I haven't looked back.'

Megan has since lowered her PBs to 17.06 for 5k, 35.46 for 10k, and 78.04 for a half marathon. She's also ran a sub-three hour marathon. She has been on the elite women's start at events including the Great South Run. 'If it wasn't for parkrun, I don't think I would have gone on to achieve these things,' she says. 'It gave me the confidence and experience I needed to push myself.'

THE KEEP FITTERS

For some parkrunners, joining is not about pushing themselves to finish high up the field but about getting a weekly dose of activity to stay fit and healthy. This exercise can be a life-saver. When Simon Graves was 49-years-old, he was told by doctors that he was at high risk of a stroke or heart attack unless he lost weight and became more active. He started attending Slimming World classes, where he lost five stone. His consultant recommended he maintain his weight loss and get some exercise by joining his local parkrun in Maidenhead. Simon was reluctant. 'I was a little nervous and thought I might not fit in. I thought parkrun was for people who belonged to running clubs,' he recalls. But once he plucked up the courage to attend, he found he had nothing to worry about as 'they cater for all levels.' Simon has now run more than 350 parkruns and volunteered. His improved fitness thanks to joining in the 5ks each week gave him the confidence to

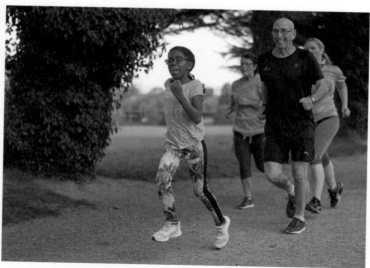

The joy of parkrun: a great way to keep fit in the outdoors

train more and take on further race distances up to the marathon. More importantly, his risk of having a heart attack has plummeted, along with his blood pressure and cholesterol. Now aged 59, parkrun is a key part of his healthy lifestyle and he hopes to inspire others by his transformation. 'Come along and have a go,' he urges those who might think they aren't fit enough to join in. You will never be last as we have parkwalkers and a tail walker who goes at the speed of the slowest person.'

Richard Elms does parkrun at Ferry Meadows in Cambridgeshire 'to keep fit and have fun' after heart surgery. 'I did my first parkrun exactly three months after I was lying on an operating table undergoing open heart surgery to replace my aortic valve,' he proudly reveals. 'I wanted to get fit again after the surgery as I used to scuba dive and cycle a lot. These sports weren't an option during my recovery period but doctors said I could follow the Couch to 5k plan. I'd never been a runner. In fact, I hated it at school, but I completed the plan, and I've now run more than 16 parkruns. I'll never set any records, after all I'm 71, but I have taken seven minutes off the time I did on my first run and my rehabilitation team are amazed by what I've achieved.'

Diane Oates also started parkrunning – at Ormskirk parkrun in Lancashire – to enhance her fitness as she ages. 'I started running parkruns in 2015 to keep me feeling young,' she says. 'I have just turned 67 and I have arthritis in my hips and my knees but I can't imagine life without it. It also helps my mental health, it's that time for you, whether you finish in 20 minutes, 30 minutes or an hour plus.'

Jane Martin, who is closing in on 250 parkruns, agrees: 'I have been a parkrunner since the very first year it started in Bushy and I simply join in to keep fit. If I've made it to a parkrun on a Saturday morning, it helps me keep a healthy mind to not waste that effort of the 5k achieved. I have been to 14 different locations and if it is a challenging course, I'll volunteer as a parkwalker, since 5k is 5k out in the fresh air no matter how you get round.'

THE DOG RUNNERS

Dogs are welcome at the vast majority of parkruns. In fact, you could say it was thanks to a dog that the whole thing started. Being tripped up by his dog when they were out running together caused the injury that sidelined Paul Sinton-Hewitt, giving him the time and motivation to organise the first time trial. However, there are some exceptions to dogs being allowed at events if a course isn't suitable for them or the landowners won't permit them – so it is always worth double-checking before you attend with your four-legged friend.

Only one dog is permitted per parkrunner and they must be on a short, handheld, non-extendable lead at all times. As dogs can be big fans of parkrun and show their passion vocally at the start, owners are asked to keep excited pets away from the pre-run briefing if they are barking loudly, so everyone else can hear what is being said.

Katherine Wilson, a self-employed glass artist, has run at more than 170 venues including Rushcliffe parkrun and Sherwood Pines parkrun, both in Nottinghamshire where she lives, with her whippets, Ripley (who sadly recently passed away) and Spider. She says: 'For me, parkrun is not the same without a dog. They get very excited at the beginning, want to say hello to everyone, and just love to run. I find it so much easier to keep going with my canine motivator with me all the time. It is also great to volunteer with your dog, particularly as a Tail Walker.'

Katherine has discovered a whole new community of dog parkrunners thanks to her involvement. She runs a Facebook group called 'parkrun dogs' where they can share their favourite dog-friendly parkruns and recommend cafes where their canines can get a sausage afterwards.

If you want to join in with your dog, Katherine recommends getting them a suitable harness to attach their lead to, rather than attaching one to a collar at their neck, as this can cause them to strain and hurt themselves. She said owners should be wary of running with them in 'very hot or cold weather', and to let them run at their own pace, stopping to sniff and have toilet breaks whenever necessary.

Carolyn Ife, who has run more than 80 parkruns including Conkers parkrun in Leicestershire, Eastleigh parkrun in Hampshire and Wimpole Estate parkrun in Cambridgeshire, with her dog, recommends 'choosing a quiet parkrun to start with' while you get used to running with your dog – and 'not worrying about finishing the first few times.'

Ellie Colman, 37, from Hampshire is another keen dog-runner who regularly partakes in parkrun tourism with her friend's husky cross, Blue. Blue has run at venues including Dorset's Upton House parkrun and Blandford parkrun, Prospect parkrun in Berkshire, Cranleigh parkrun in Surrey, Cannock Chase parkrun in Staffordshire and Itchen Valley Country parkrun in Hampshire, to name but a few. Ellie, who is a specialist speech and language therapist, says: 'I really love taking part with a dog at parkrun because it encourages a lot more people to chat to me. I think

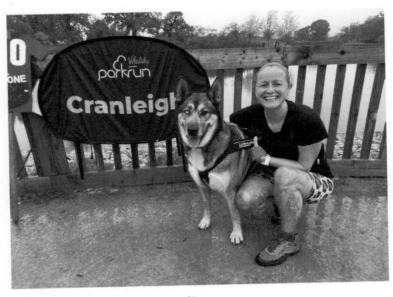

Dog runner Ellie Colman with husky cross, Blue

DID YOU KNOW?

Incidents of collisions with dogs taking part have fallen since parkrun enforced the handheld lead rule.

having the dog opens up conversation more easily than when I'm on my own. I've always felt very welcomed at the venues we've done together. I think he's a good distraction for people too when they might be finding it a bit tough to keep going, and he often encourages children along. He always gets lots of attention and people giving him treats after!'

She adds: 'If you're going to take your dog to a parkrun, I would suggest checking out the different event pages first and looking at what the courses are like. I prefer to go to ones with grass or gravel tracks as it's better for Blue. I also tend to opt for less crowded ones and with few loops as these can be more congested. You could start by walking or volunteering to introduce your dog if they aren't used to running with others. Most importantly go and have fun with your dog!'

If you do join in, note you can't use a lead that attaches around your waist. parkrun banned this type of harness in 2022 due to concerns over participants' safety. It claimed trips and falls were more likely with this type of lead, especially as owners might have less control over the direction their dog runs in. The ban has proved controversial as many dog owners prefer to run with their dog this way, and now feel they can no longer participate. parkrun states on its website that anyone with an assistance dog who needs to run with one on a waist harness can still do so, but they need to apply to their head office first for an exception.

Carolyn said she 'much prefers' to run with her dog on a waist harness, but understands why the decision was made as 'fast out of control dogs on a waist harness can be a real hazard.'

Ellie said she was initially 'upset' about the rule change, as she feared she wouldn't be able to run with Blue any more and they would both miss out on doing something they love together. She has been able to use a handheld lead, but hasn't found it easy as

Blue is so strong. She worries this might stop other dog runners from taking part, which is at odds with parkrun's inclusivity ethos.

'In particular from my experience the rule change has impacted more upon women who run with larger dogs,' she points out. 'It has meant a lot of people have been excluded from the community because they can only run with their dog using the waist harness. It would have been a good time for parkrun to work with the professional bodies who are expert in this area to promote how to run with your dog safely and to encourage all participants to be courteous and more aware of each other. I've only ever had positive interactions with other parkrunners about Blue, and I think dogs being part of the community really is important to a lot of people.'

THE BUGGY RUNNERS

Lack of childcare can be a major barrier to exercise for many parents – so being able to join in a parkrun with a baby or child in a buggy is a boon. parkrun encourages the use of pushchairs, prams and running buggies but points out that not all courses are 'appropriate' – for example if they have super steep hills. So 'it is the responsibility of the adult participant to determine the suitability of the course', and whether they can safely push a child around the route. The other stipulations are that you are not allowed to run with both a dog and a buggy, or with an additional child on a 'buggy board'. Running buggies where the child is pulled along behind the parent in a trailer attached to their waist are also banned for safety reasons.

Running buggy manufacturers recommend babies should not be pushed at speed in their pushchairs until they are at least six months old, and have the neck strength to support their own heads, because of the potential impact on their growing bodies. However, this doesn't mean a parent has to wait until their baby is old enough to run with to take part. If they wish, they can walk a parkrun with their newborn lying flat in a pram. Once a baby is

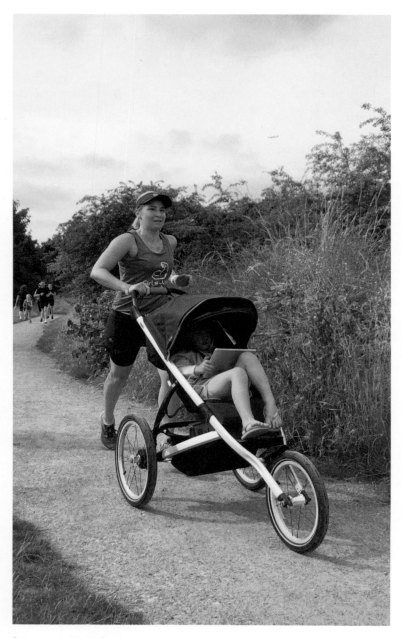

Buggy runner Wendy Rumble

old enough and a parent wants to run with them, it is advisable to get a running buggy suitable for pushing at a faster pace, for both the comfort and safety of the passenger, and to make it easier to push. This includes having a fixed front wheel, large inflatable tyres, a handbrake and a wrist strap. Wendy Rumble set up a business and Facebook group called The Original Buggy Runners during her maternity leave in 2015 to encourage parents to be active with their young ones. She said mums, dads and guardians should embrace the opportunity to join in a parkrun for their mental and physical health. 'Parenting can be really lonely and is mentally tough. By buggy running at parkrun parents can connect with others in their community, while also giving themselves a boost through exercise,' she says. 'Over the years I've heard numerous stories from single parents, parents who do shift work, and partners of those in the military who couldn't fit in any exercise if they didn't have a running buggy. The buzz that you get from being outdoors in nature, being with others and moving your body is amazing.' Wendy regularly pushed her daughters in a running buggy at Maidenhead parkrun in Berkshire, and has plenty of tips for those who want to follow in her tyre tracks: 'Some people are nervous about going to parkrun to buggy run but don't put any pressure on yourself as you get used to it, it's a different kind of run,' she says. 'If your little one can't settle you can just stop. But in my experience, they do settle – often falling asleep – or when they are older chatting about what they can see. Some people play music to entertain them, some people give snacks to older kids. The rain cover can be comforting if it is windy as it keeps some warmth in too.' When it comes to manoeuvring during the run, she advises: 'Line up on the start line at the right place for your pace to reduce the amount of overtaking you have to do. Then if you do overtake, shout "buggy on your right" to make people aware. It's amazing how encouraging people are, I would always get heaps of comments as I ran around about being super mum and could they hitch a ride on the buggy!'

DID YOU KNOW?

Olympic medallist Josh Kerr grew up racing parkruns with his family in Scotland, and once clocked sub 23 minutes while pushing his nephew in a running buggy.

Now Wendy's daughters are older, they still love joining in parkrun. But now they run on their own two feet as regular junior parkrunners, proof that exposing young children to exercise can make it a part of normal life for them.

Heather Hann, 38, from Hertfordshire, found buggy-running at parkrun a lifeline after she became a mum for the first time. 'Running had always been a big part of my life but when I first had a baby, I wondered if I would ever run again,' she recalls. 'I had found pregnancy and labour physically and mentally draining, and lack of childcare meant I could no longer go to my running club's evening sessions. As a result, I found motherhood to be pretty isolating at times and I missed my old running life. It was then a friend offered me a running buggy and I was hooked – it gave me the freedom to run again.' She started doing her nearest parkrun in St Albans with her baby in the running buggy, running alongside her husband. Once Heather had regained her fitness, she decided to take on a big new race challenge. In 2021, she broke the Guinness World Record for the fastest 10k pushing a pram. 'I wanted to help parents realise that running goals don't have to fall by the wayside when you are looking after young children. You can get out there with a running buggy and you may even find you completely smash your PBs!' she says. 'I hope I can inspire others. It's amazing to see so many buggy runners at my local parkrun receiving so much support and encouragement.'

Matt Coyne, 42, a father-of-three from Sussex is another avid buggy parkrunner. He's done nearly 100 pushing either a single or double running buggy, mostly at venues on the South coast including Seaford Beach parkrun, Peacehaven parkrun, Hove Promenade parkrun, and Lancing Beach Green parkrun. Once on holiday, he even took on the infamous Woolacombe Dunes parkrun course in Devon pushing his daughter in a buggy (read more about this challenging parkrun in Chapter Seven).

Matt, who is the founder of a free running group called RunPals, says he loves that parkrun allows people to join in pushing buggies, as all the family can experience the benefits.

'Being a parent shouldn't mean giving up on activities and hobbies that you used to enjoy before having children,' he says. 'parkrun provides an opportunity for parents like myself to continue pursuing their passion for running, or generally being outside and active, while also spending quality time with their little ones. It also sets a great example for children to see their parents being active and partici-pating in a community event. It helps promote a healthy lifestyle from an early age and shows the importance of exercise and physical activity for families. Since starting out in parkrun together, my now five-year-old has been my number one run pal. I started with her in the buggy when she was six months, and when she was about two, she would start off in the buggy, hop out and run for a bit, then jump back in when she was tired. Now she mostly runs or walks with me. We talk for hours when out together on our adventures and those memories will last for a lifetime – hers and mine.'

Matt adds that regularly attending parkrun has led to his family making many new friends.

'I would say it's not just the running that's had a positive impact, but the friends we have made and the benefits those connections have on our mental health and wellbeing,' he explains. 'Since my pal, Jon, introduced me to parkrun some years ago, we have made so many friends through this community and to quote another pal Leigh, "I never thought I'd make new friends in my forties". parkrun has introduced us to not just adult friends but families that are connected through a passion of being outside and running together each Saturday morning. It is a great way to enjoy the Great Outdoors whether you walk, run, or wheel.'

For anyone considering joining in with a buggy, Matt says: 'Just do it. The hardest thing to do with buggy running is starting. Just turn up and give it a go. Sure, it's not all rosy. It can be tough on some courses or those with a tonne of people on narrow paths, so choose a nice, flat course to begin with and just take your time. Remove all expectations of time. Remember, as much as it may take time for you to get used to buggy running, it may also take your co-pilot some time to adjust too. The initial novelty of doing it may wear off soon if they are toddler stage and they may just not want to go with you at all. Be patient and encouraging with them, and enjoy the experience of sharing your love for parkrun with your little one.'

THE FAMILY RUNNERS

parkrun is a family affair for many, who love to join in with their relatives. As well as the buggy runners, there are those who enjoy running with their older children and other relatives. This is the case for Karen Sheard, 50, a PA, and her husband, Richard, 53, a director of engineering, who find parkrun an ideal way to spend time with their sons aged 18, 15 and 11.

'Now that two of my sons are teenagers, and none of them are particularly sporty, we love the fact parkrun brings us all together for an hour every weekend, doing an activity that is physical and outside in the fresh air,' Karen says. 'I love the inclusivity of parkrun – this is especially helpful when you have three sons who often need some encouragement to run! My youngest and I jointly ran our 50th on the same day, and I've since gone on to run more than 130.' They mostly participate in Hertfordshire events, but have also taken part while on holiday in Cornwall and the Peak District. As well as running, their sons have volunteered regularly at parkrun as part of their Duke of Edinburgh Awards.

Karen's brother-in-laws are also big parkrun fans and sharing their parkrun adventures brings the brothers together, even though they now live in different parts of the country, one in Harwell, Oxford, and the other in North Wales. 'Each Saturday without fail the brothers

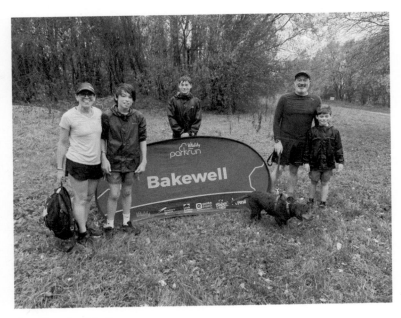

Karen Sheard and family

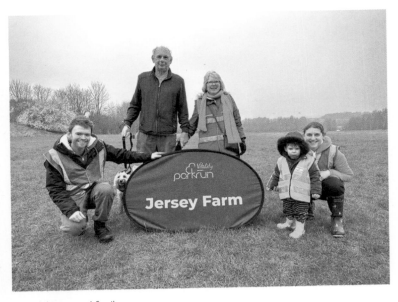

Laura Johnston and family

send a photo to each other from whichever parkrun they are running or volunteering at, with a little report on how it has gone.'

Running with partners and children is not the only family benefit of parkrun. Sometimes it starts families. Laura Johnston, 34, a teacher from the town of Harpenden in Hertfordshire, and Alex had known each other since they were seven, but lost touch when they went to university. They met again at Heartwood Forest parkrun in 2017. A few years later, at Jersey Farm parkrun on Laura's birthday in 2021, Alex proposed. 'If parkrun didn't exist it's likely Alex and I wouldn't have got together,' Laura says. 'We now have a two-year-old son, Charlie, who loves parkrun and can't wait to go each week. parkrun was one of his first words.' Laura and Alex have pushed Charlie around numerous events in a running buggy and he loves looking out for his grandmother marshalling on 'Nanny corner' and for Alex's mum, Joanne Martin, who is also a frequent volunteer and runner. Laura's aunt, Maxine Slade, also regularly joins in. Laura says: 'For us, parkrun is a chance to catch up with friends and family whilst doing something healthy and enjoyable. It's great that we can all be involved whether running or volunteering and then all go to the cafe together afterwards.'

Iain Hall, 62, a retired car dealer from Stockton-on-Tees, also gets involved with the different generations of his family, who are racking up the milestones along with the speedy PBs.

Iain first started parkrunning in his late forties. He completed his very first parkrun in 2008 at Albert parkrun, in Middlesbrough, when it was one of only nine parkruns in the world and was still called a time trial. Someone suggested he join in after he gained a charity place to do the Great North Run. Before parkrun, he only ran at the gym on a treadmill. 'After that very first run – which I finished in 21.12 – I was hooked. I couldn't wait until the following week to do it again. This has stayed with me and now I have done nearly 700 at 251 locations and got my time down to 18:38. I enjoy the support, encouragement and social aspect of parkrun, which led me to entering other races in many distances of 5 miles up to marathons.'

Joyfully, Iain has passed the parkrun bug onto his children and grandchildren. 'I knew my children would love it too, so I encouraged my son, James, then 22, to join me for my second one,' he recalls. 'He's since completed 264 with a PB of 18.29, and he's passed the passion down to the next generation as he now takes his children, Isaac, 11, and Isla, eight, along. My daughter, Rachael, now 33, then did her first parkrun in 2013, and is now approaching 400 parkruns with a PB of 21:12. Her children Alfie, 14, and Jack, 11, are also parkrunners.

Iain even converted his wife, Ann, to becoming a parkrunner, even though when she met him in 2012, she told him: 'Iain, I'll come and support you at your parkruns, but I'll never run. I don't even run for a bus.'

Ann, 57, decided to volunteer instead and after seeing the participants of varied abilities, ages, and sizes taking part, she thought to herself: 'If they can do it, so can I.' She followed a Couch to 5k plan and ran her first parkrun in under 40 minutes. She's since got her PB down to 30:11, run a half marathon, and continues to volunteer at parkrun and junior parkrun, along with Iain. April 2024 was a big milestone moment for the family as they celebrated Rachael's 400th

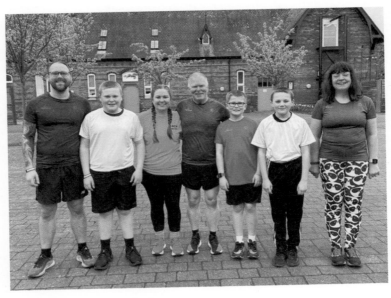

Iain Hall and his parkrunning family

and Jack's 50th on the same day. Iain says he loves how his grandchildren are growing up as parkrunners alongside their grandparents and parents. 'parkrun means everything to us, we plan our family holidays so we can visit different locations.'

THE MILESTONE MARKERS

Making a milestone is special to many parkrunners and it motivates them to attend week in, week out. Louise Thompson, 48, a Senior Content Designer from West Yorkshire started her tally in July 2010 and is currently working her way towards her 500th. 'The milestones mean a lot to me because they're a real mark of perseverance. It doesn't matter how fast or slow you are, everyone can earn a T-shirt and wear it with pride,' she says. 'Reaching my first milestone was a really proud moment. My 100th was memorable as I ran dressed as a Christmas tree as it was that time of year and a work friend had shown up with a 100 banner that she'd made.' Louise's milestones mean so much to her, she jokes that if her house was on fire, she'd run in to save her 100 milestone jacket. parkrun has become 'the highlight' of her week – she sees so many friends there and has visited places she may never have gone to otherwise. She always celebrates her milestones (official and unofficial) at her home event, Wakefield Thornes parkrun, in Wakefield, along with her running club buddies from Rodillian Runners. 'The club has a great tradition of turning out to support our runners' milestones and I love seeing everyone in club shirts having a great morning, and a cafe trip after, in the true spirit of parkrun.'

Katherine Tomlinson, from Yorkshire, is aiming for a century by setting herself the challenge of running 100 parkruns by the time she is 40 years old. 'In order to this, I can't miss a week for seven months,' she says. 'I set the challenge to motivate me to go even when I'm not feeling 100 percent. If I am genuinely too ill to attend then I will miss it and change my goal, or I have the option to walk it instead of run. I've made some silly excuses in the past to avoid going so this challenge will stop me from doing that, as I know I always feel better physically and most importantly mentally after joining in.'

Jaqui McGee from Middlesbrough can relate to this post parkrun high which she gets by chasing milestones and visiting new parkrun venues. So far she has done more than 81 parkruns at 51 locations with a tourist streak of 36. She has completed the 'Alphabet challenge' – running a parkrun starting with every letter of the alphabet – and recently joined the 'world tourist club' by parkrunning in four or more different countries. She says: 'I'm motivated by the post parkrun feeling of achievement, visiting different places, and stepping outside my comfort zone.'

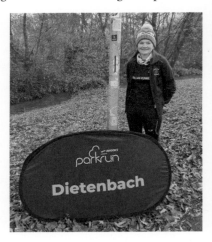

Milestone runner Louise Thompson

Chris Dyke is another self-confessed 'milestone nerd'. 'I did way too much planning in 2022 to ensure that I hit my 250th run and 250th volunteering on the same run by joining in as a pacer,' he says. 'I live in London so I can visit a variety without having to travel very far, so I have also reached 50 different events. I'm now on 300 runs and 326 volunteering. Getting to 500 seems a long way off but it will be fun to keep working towards it. I love everything about parkrun, it is a great social fixture.'

Reaching a milestone is also a big deal for South Londoner Debbie Williams and her friends who celebrate both the official 50th, 100th, and 250th and unofficial 150th, 200th, and 300th ones they reach, usually by donning fancy dress. Debbie, 57, who works

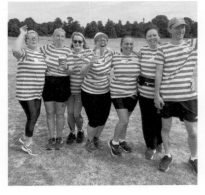

Debbie Williams (centre, wearing a hat) on a Where's Wally-themed parkrun with friends

in administration, has done 167 in total at 69 different locations and volunteered 50 times. She says: 'Milestones are massive as they are a recognition of your progress. There's about 16 in my running group – Croydon Crazy Crew – and when it's a special milestone that person decides on the parkrun and dress up theme. We've had "Where's Wally?", onesies, ducks and 80s themes to name but a few. Dressing up brings extra joy to the parkrun.'

THE PARTICIPANTS WITH DISABILITIES

In 2016, parkrun launched the PROVE project in England to widen access to those with disabilities. Volunteer Outreach Ambassadors were recruited to encourage people to participate as runners, walkers or volunteers, and set up private support groups on Facebook that people could join to access further advice, such as those with diabetes and autism. At the events themselves, there are specific volunteer roles to help those with disabilities. For example, you can volunteer as a guide runner to help those who are visually impaired or need assistance to get around a course safely. And there's a volunteer role to sign the pre-run and first timers briefing for the benefit of attendees who may be deaf or hard of hearing. Wheelchair users are welcome at parkruns, but parkrun HQ says the suitability of courses

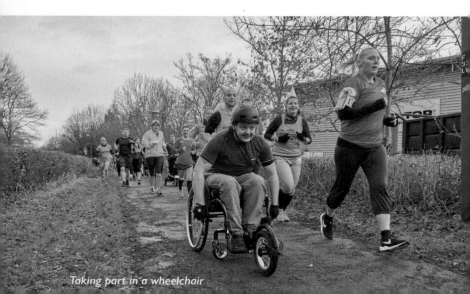

Taking part in a wheelchair

will vary and so participation will 'depend on the skill, experience, and confidence of the wheelchair user'. It urges them to check with the event team before attending if they have any concerns over the route.

Charlotte Laitner, 24, who has Down Syndrome, has found a place at parkrun where she can exercise and have fun. She enjoyed running but felt the local athletics club where her sisters trained 'didn't feel like the sort of place I could go'. She once thought parkrun wouldn't be suitable for her either, so put off going. 'When I run I like to take my time and go quite slowly at first,' she explains. 'I used to think that everyone else at

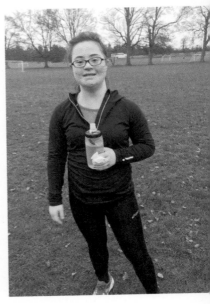

Charlotte Laitner at a parkrun

parkrun was so fast so I didn't want to do it.' But with the encouragement of her running mum, Nicky, Charlotte gave it a chance. 'At first, I was nervous about going but the people there were really nice and I found lots of people that I knew, including friends from my Special Olympics group, and that made me happy. My family were there to cheer me on and the marshals were really encouraging.' Completing the 5k gave Charlotte the confidence to push herself further, and she went on to do a half marathon, raising money for charity in the process. She continues to do parkrun and loves how it makes her feel happy and healthy. 'Get out of bed and come down, the marshals will cheer you on,' she urges others. 'It doesn't matter if you are slow. You will feel so proud of yourself at the end.'

Jethro Offemaria, 34, from Hemel Hempstead, who has autism, plucked up the courage to join in a parkrun at the end of 2023, and he didn't regret it. 'I have always loved running so I was curious about parkrun. I decided to go for the first time after I left a mental health hospital. I was nervous about going but I had huge support from

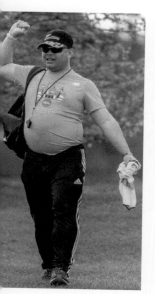

parkrun enthusiast Jethro Offemaria (Graham Smith)

fellow runners at Spider Runners – a running community I am part of. I jogged and walked and it went really well.' He has now done many more parkruns as well as volunteering. 'It motivates me to exercise and it is a stress-buster so it is very good for my mental health. I've also volunteered as a marshal numerous times and I love cheering everyone on. Seeing others running and walking motivates me. It's definitely an autistic-friendly event so I recommend it to others. Register for a barcode and come along!'

Dijana White, 48, agrees. She's seen the health and happiness of her son transform thanks to joining in California Country Park parkrun near their home in Finchampstead, Berkshire.

'In 2019, my husband, Olly and I started taking it in turns to do the parkrun with our daughter, Hannah, while the other looked after our son Luka, then 13, who has autism and sensory processing difficulties,' she says. 'We started to wonder: "Could Luka manage 5k, even if he walks it?" We knew parkrun has such a family-oriented environment, if we ever wanted to give him a chance to do it, then this was the place. We decided to give it a go and took our dog, Freddy, with us for support.'

'We never expected what happened next,' she recalls. 'Luka not only ran the full 5k but afterwards said, "I love it and want to do it again!" From then on, parkrun became our Saturday morning thing as it was so accessible, friendly and accepting. We realised how important exercise was for Luka and his sensory needs so following the parkrun success, we gained the confidence to enrol him in other sports.' Luka is now an all round athlete. He's a great swimmer and competes in galas, loves tennis, is a member of a football club, and holds a purple belt in Taijutsu. He was the first child from his SEN school to run in the Berkshire Schools Cross Country Championship, where he managed to qualify and run to represent the county. 'We're part of our lovely local Finch Coasters running club and have done 10ks to half marathon races as a family', says Dijana. Now aged 18 and more than 120 parkruns later, Luka has become stronger and faster with a PB of 20.28. 'We are currently looking into different exciting races we can do together. This has all happened because of parkrun. It hasn't just had a huge impact on Luka but on us as well and our mental health. parkrun is a big part of our weekly routine and our social life. I love to empower other parents of SEN children to have a go, as it could make a huge impact on your child and yourselves. Thanks to our parkrun community and our running friends, we can look to Luka's future with a more positive lens.'

parkrun has also allowed Damian Tancred, 49, a gym instructor and personal trainer from Sydney, Australia, to have a more positive outlook after he was diagnosed with Multiple sclerosis (MS) 10 years ago.

'Looking back, I had MS symptoms from the age of 24,' he explains. 'My symptoms got progressively worse over a long period of time. This included blurred vision, spasticity in both legs, poor balance, poor coordination, brain fog, daily fatigue and heat sensitivity to hot or cold weather. Both extremes exacerbate my condition. MS is a progressive disease of the central nervous system that can affect the brain and spinal cord. There is no cure but there is medication to slow the degeneration.'

Prior to his diagnosis, Damian had been a talented runner over middle distances, particularly 800m and 1500m, and he feared his condition would mean he could never enjoy running again.

'As my MS got worse, I saw a drop in my athletic performance, for example from 15 minutes for 5k to 25 minutes, with a large

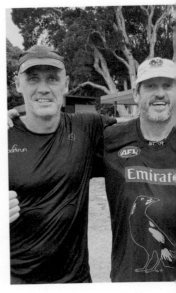

Damian Tancred (left) at a parkrun with a friend.

effort required. This made me feel really low as I missed my old athletic life,' he recalls. 'So I thank God for the invention of parkrun as it rejuvenated my hobby. I did my first back in 2015 and I have since done more than 125 at various locations in Australia. I know I am never going to run a PB but old habits die hard and I still try to run them competitively. I'm also hooked on reaching the milestones. I loved getting my hands on the beautiful purple shirt after reaching 25, and now I'm looking forward to getting the green one for 250. I thought running was all over for me after my MS diagnosis but parkrun has given me a new lease of life.' He adds: 'For me, it's not just about the running, I enjoy having a coffee with my friends afterwards too. It is also so great to be able to travel the country and know there will be a parkrun somewhere nearby. The phrase I regularly hear after a parkrun is "that's the best way to start the weekend". I couldn't agree more.'

THE FIRST TIMERS

Going to a parkrun for the first time can be a big step, particularly for someone who doesn't consider themself to be a runner. This is why parkrun have taken measures – such as removing the course record stats from their websites and introducing parkwalking volunteers – to encourage newcomers. Vicky Yaxley, a mum in her early forties, admits she was once too nervous to join in her local parkrun as she thought it would be 'too competitive', so she put off going for years. She changed her mind when she had a look at the weekly results and saw there was a huge range of times. 'I then posted on my local parkrun's event Facebook page and the reply was so welcoming and helpful that I took the plunge,' she recalls. 'In February 2024, I did it with my 10-year-old son and it was amazing. There was such a mix of people and just the friendliest and supportive vibe. The volunteers high-fived my son as he made his way round. I'm now looking forward to going again and improving my time.'

Jude Wilson, 60, from South Devon, understands how many first timers might feel apprehensive about being too slow to take part, but says in her experience there is no need to worry. 'I was post-meno-pausal and in a very stressful job as a residential conveyancing solicitor when I first tried Torbay Velopark parkrun. I decided I wanted to get a bit fitter and having done Race For Life years ago I thought I would give it a go. I pitched up and walked and jogged around. No one mocked me for being slow, and people were supportive and kind,' she reassures. 'I get that there are the "racing snakes" who I could never hope to get anywhere near in time. But mostly I believe that people do it because it's fun and no pressure. My husband has now started volunteering and we've made friends with the core

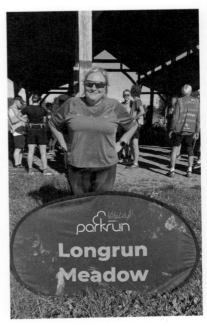

First timer Jude Wilson

team. It has been just lovely for both my mental and physical health. I tell all my friends they should be doing it.'

Mum of three Susie Faulkner is another recent convert having attended her local event, Market Harborough parkrun in Leicester-shire, for the first time in 2024.

She said: 'I'd joined a local running club called Great Bowden Runners to keep fit and the coach, Lily Canter, suggested it would be good training, and another opportunity to run with others, to join in a parkrun. I'd heard of it before, and have taken my children to the junior parkrun once or twice, but due to their various clubs/activities at weekends, I'd never been able to make one myself. In January 2024, I finally seized my chance. I was more intrigued and excited than nervous before I went, and I knew a friend who goes regularly would meet up with me at the end. On the day, it exceeded all my expectations! It was such a lovely atmosphere. I loved that

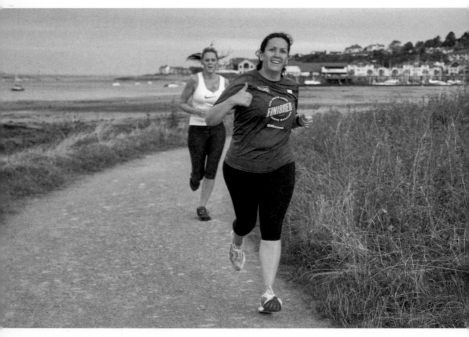

Spectacular scenery is one of the big draws of parkrun

some people were a bit competitive and others were just happy to be out doing it. You could take exactly what you wanted from it, which you can't get anywhere else. My finish time was 27.36 which I was very happy with and it left me keen to do more – I like the look of the T-shirts you get when you've done 25/50/100 parkruns. I just wish family life wasn't so busy and I could disappear every Saturday morning to do parkrun!'

If you're still not convinced, then let Conan McGhee, 24, from Glasgow, inspire you. He has a rare cancerous tumour and was encouraged to join in parkrun by his nurse to enhance his health. She recommended he attend with a '5k Your Way' support group (read more about this community-based initiative in Chapter Five). Conan says: 'I was reluctant at first. When I was younger I was a member of an athletics club so I know runners can be competitive in wanting to beat their PBs. I worried I might get in their way if

I was walking, and it might make me speed up and struggle with my own breathing.'

He adds: 'I'm also quite an anti-social person and I can feel quite awkward when meeting groups of people I don't know. So parkrun didn't appeal to me. My girlfriend, Milly, is quite the opposite and can talk and get on with almost everyone. So she pushed me to at least try it and see what it was like.'

With the support of Milly and the 5KYW group, Conan walked around Elder Park parkrun in Glasgow and was pleasantly surprised that all his reservations were wrong.

'I loved that I could do it my way at my own pace,' he recalls. 'The support from the volunteers, other runners and the 5KYW ambassadors along the way was really motivating. Crossing the finish line was quite an emotional experience. A few months before, I'd had a sternotomy to remove some of a tumour that was suffocating my heart causing heart failure. Before my surgery, I couldn't walk the length of my house and really struggled with my breathing. I was at risk of being bedbound. So, for me to complete a 5k, even though I walked it, without needing to stop and without struggling with my breathing was a major achievement.' He has done several more parkruns and his health has improved greatly. 'I've gone from being someone who couldn't really walk much at all to being able to complete 5ks, walking faster each time. I'm still undergoing treatment and parkrun motivates me to keep walking to help improve my health and well-being. To anyone reading this who is nervous about going for the first time and thinks it's not for them, I say just try it once because you'll probably be really surprised.'

THE WALKERS

Walking has long been acceptable at parkruns and a tail-walking volunteer always strolls at the back. However, in 2022, a parkrun survey found that some people still didn't feel comfortable attending

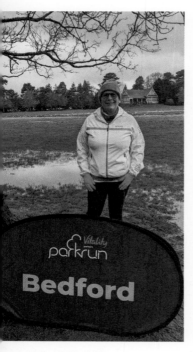

Walker Debbie Niblett

if they weren't running. They felt they couldn't join in unless they were fitter and faster. In a bid to counter this view and boost their numbers after a dip in attendance following the Covid-19 pandemic, parkrun launched 'parkwalk' to encourage people to attend parkrun as walkers. It also created the volunteer role of 'parkwalker' – someone who attends and walks the whole way (in front of the tail walker) to encourage and represent other walkers. parkrun said the campaign was a means of giving people 'permission' to walk at their events, and letting them know you can never be too slow to take part. Liz Burkey is one of the people who has become a parkrun convert thanks to parkwalk and she's since completed more than 50 in the UK and Europe. 'I started in 2023 as a walker who wanted to start running,' she recalls. 'parkwalk definitely helped me feel that it was OK to be slower than 30 minutes, and that I wouldn't be holding everyone up. I still walk more than I run but I am getting faster and enjoy the tourism aspect of parkrun – seeing new places and completing challenges.'

Debbie Niblett, 57, from Coventry, also says she isn't a runner, but parkrun has become a Saturday morning staple after a friend told her she could walk.

'I didn't know you could walk – I thought it was for runners,' she recalls. After a girls' weekend away where they all had great fun walking or running at Wollaton Hall parkrun in Nottingham, she became a convert. 'Some of us wanted to continue going so we looked into completing challenges to keep us motivated. We're now supporting one another each week, having a real good laugh and

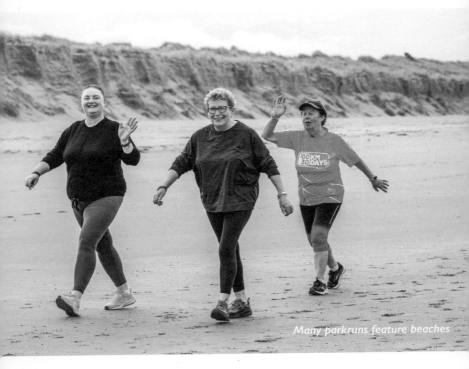

Many parkruns feature beaches

getting out to different venues as tourists,' she says. 'I'm still not a runner – I don't like going out running in the week on my own – but I do love the atmosphere of a parkrun. My time is improving and I'm managing to run more than walk. Saturdays are now built around parkrun in the morning and we'll often head for a coffee after. Now I would encourage anyone to join whatever their ability. We met an amazing woman called Margaret at Brueton parkrun in Solihull who has done more than 400 – and she's just turned 90. She does it with a walking frame – what a legend. And I've also seen someone at Oaklands parkrun in Birmingham in a wheelchair. Walk, run, hop or crawl. Just do it. The buzz is amazing. The volunteers are amazing. And best of all I get to spend a morning with some good friends.'

Of course no parkrun is able to happen without volunteers, while parkrun tourists are also a common sight. Read on for more on them in Chapters Three and Six respectively...

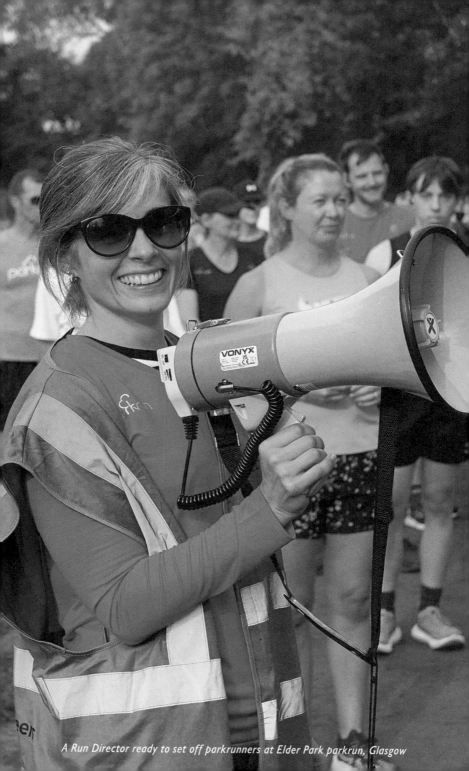

A Run Director ready to set off parkrunners at Elder Park parkrun, Glasgow

CHAPTER THREE
THE HIGH-VIS HEROES

Without the dedication of the high-vis heroes, aka volunteers, parkrun would not have kept going for two decades or expanded around the world. It is thanks to people giving their time for free that events take place. Some parkrunners love to alternate volunteering with running or walking the course. Other volunteers never actively join in but love to help out. Some volunteer roles, such as pacing and event set-up, mean you can both run/walk and volunteer on the same day.

Often parkruns might be short of volunteers ahead of an event so can appeal for people to come forward on social media, but parkrun insists there should never be any pressure on people to step forward.

'It is absolutely our belief that volunteering should be done simply for the pleasure of helping out and for the benefits that are gained from doing so,' it states on its website. 'There should be no pressure for parkrunners to volunteer at events. While the roster does need to be filled each week, we ask people to volunteer when they would like to, and for event teams to create an environment where people feel welcomed, included and supported.'

parkrun adds that: 'Volunteering at parkrun is an equal form of participation, where the act of volunteering itself is the reward.'

This means volunteers who might never join in as a runner or walker can still have their own barcodes to log the number of times they have volunteered, and like participants, they can work towards milestones of 50, 100, 250 etc and buy associated merchandise to celebrate. parkrun started recording the number of volunteers at each event in the results from 2008, and these stats can be found in the 'event history' lists on each event page.

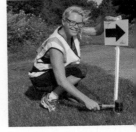

Preparing the course

BENEFITS OF VOLUNTEERING

Numerous studies have shown that volunteering your time and energy can boost your mental health. Knowing you are helping others causes your brain to release the happiness hormone, dopamine, which makes you feel good. Volunteering – particularly at a parkrun – is a means of being sociable, meeting new people, getting out and about, and gaining a sense of belonging. This reduces isolation and loneliness, which in turn can prevent and reduce mental illnesses such as depression. If you live alone, a parkrun provides a chance every Saturday to go and mix with others and feel part of your community. Volunteering has been found to reduce stress levels, and it can also lift self-confidence by giving someone a sense of purpose and making them feel valued. Not only that, volunteering can help develop skills that can be beneficial in other areas of your

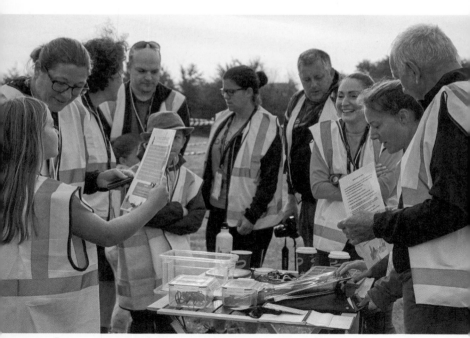

From course set up to finishing tokens: Volunteers have lots of jobs to do

life. For example, by taking on a Run Director role at a parkrun, someone could develop the confidence and skills needed to take on a more managerial role in their career. For young people, it could give them some experience of how to work with others and problem-solve before they enter a workplace.

Research has shown the benefits of volunteering aren't just mental, but physical too. A study carried out in 2013 found that volunteering can reduce blood pressure in those aged over 50. Another found that people who volunteered lived longer than those who didn't. It is thought this is because volunteering made people more active, and more likely to use their brains, keeping their bodies and minds sharper when ageing. In 2019, parkrun did its own research into the benefits felt by its volunteers. More than 60,000 responded. Of those, 84 percent said volunteering at parkrun made them feel happier. Chrissie Wellington, a former world Ironman champion and now parkrun's Global Head of Health and Wellbeing, said of these findings: 'It is clear that volunteering is an incredibly positive activity in its own right, with the greatest health and well-being gains being seen by the thousands of people who volunteer at parkrun. People may be motivated by altruistic factors, but this research supports our belief that volunteering at parkrun benefits the individual in a range of ways, as well as the community they are part of.'

'WHY WE VOLUNTEER'

Beatrice, 48, and Des Merrigan, a married couple, volunteer (and run) regularly at Black Park parkrun, Buckinghamshire. Des said: 'It's a good way to ensure we get out the door on Saturdays. It is lovely to meet up with various friends we have made over the years. In a strange way, it doesn't really matter about the weather any more, as we will go regardless, although it is always nicer if it's not raining! I mainly enjoy volunteering because of the banter with the other volunteers, there is always time for a chat amongst the team. It is nice when the runners thank you for volunteering.

It really is a great way to spend a couple of hours, meet people and make their (and your) day by making them smile. You will go home feeling like you have made the world a better place.' Beatrice agrees: 'Volunteering is about giving something back to the community. They say volunteering makes you feel good and I can 100 percent relate to that.'

Lucy Harrison has volunteered more than 217 times in various roles at Holkham parkrun, set in the grounds of a stately home in north Norfolk. 'I'm Event Director at Holkham, and also carry out the Run Director and any other roles needed,' she says. 'I like being at the start/finish line to see everyone as they come back so barcode scanning or handing out finish tokens are my favourite roles. I wouldn't be anywhere else on a Saturday morning – a few hours with a great group of people in a stunning location – what's not to love?'

Filitsia Rockas agrees and has volunteered at numerous parkrun venues around the world in a variety of roles. 'I really recommend volunteering when you can,' she says. 'I enjoy volunteering at parkrun as it is a good way to support your local community, get active and get out the house. I love to see participants strive towards achieving their goals and milestones.'

Danny O'Reilly, 39, regularly volunteers at Chester parkrun, Cheshire, along with his daughter, Gracie, three. 'Gracie and I have been volunteering at Chester parkrun for almost three years since she was around six-months-old,' he says. 'In those early days she'd be found napping in the pram, today she's still the youngest on the roster, but comfortably the most enthusiastic volunteer, regularly in fancy dress as a witch or Disney princess and doling out as many high-fives and "well-dones" as she can. We have volunteered 51 times, including once at Sherwood Pines parkrun

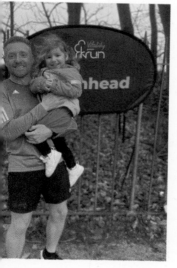

Volunteers Danny and Gracie O'Reilly

in Nottinghamshire when we were on holiday and eagerly awaiting the delivery of our latest milestone tees.' Danny, a copywriter, is passionate about volunteering at parkrun because he 'loves parkrun and what it does for communities, physical and mental health. I'm also very lucky to have run lots of courses too, so it's important to me to give back by volunteering as often as possible,' he says. 'And what I really love is spending time with my daughter at parkrun, watching her grow in confidence, engaging with the runners and seeing exercise as something normal and for everyone. She'll be four before the end of 2024 and we can't wait to take-on junior parkrun.'

Volunteering at parkrun has given Karla Gregory 'a new purpose and focus in life' after she struggled with her health. 'Previously you might have been cut off from a community as a result of a health condition, but with parkrun, you can keep in contact with like minded people, and those who run/walk and appreciate being outside,' she says. For others, volunteering allows them to stay in contact with their running community while resting an injury. This was the case for Alison Parris, 57, who started volunteering at Lalor parkrun, Australia, when she was unable to run. 'I fell off a horse and damaged my ankle so I was out of action for 18 months. This is when I started volunteering on a more regular basis. Having friends pick me up, take me to parkrun, then to breakfast and home again was a godsend! I could escape the house and still be involved with my club, Lalor Running Club. Now I continue to volunteer in various roles including RD. Our parkrun operates on a minimum of volunteers as we can't always get enough post-pandemic so most of my club volunteer regularly to keep it going each week.'

Diana Barraclough first discovered the joy of parkrun volunteering back in 2016 after going along to cheer her husband on while he was

DID YOU KNOW?

According to a parkrun survey, 98 percent of their volunteers feel valued by the parkrun community, and 97 percent say their experience was easy.

running at Doncaster's Sandall Park parkrun. 'Then I started going every week and cheered on everyone,' she recalls. 'I decided to try volunteering and I loved it! I started volunteering at the parkrun and junior parkrun regularly. I also started running in 2019 but it is the volunteering that's my passion. It's all so rewarding. The friends I have gained through doing this is amazing.'

Julie Bayliss, another volunteer, says she feels volunteering makes her feel like she is making a difference by helping people feel welcome and showing them that parkrun is for all.

'I am a huge parkrun fan,' she adds. 'I have volunteered 396 times and I can't wait to reach my 500 volunteer milestone. Through volunteering at parkrun, I have made great friends and learnt new skills too.'

THE PARKRUN CODE FOR VOLUNTEERS AT A GLANCE

- Volunteer for the love of it
- Treat everyone as a friend
- Be kind and respectful
- Unite as a team
- Be reliable, responsible and attentive
- Be helpful and enthusiastic
- Respect our principles
- Do your best

WHAT VOLUNTEER ROLES ARE THERE?

There are many volunteer roles that can be filled, but not all of them are essential for a parkrun to go ahead. The compulsory roles, often filled by what is known the 'core team' are:

Event Director: Each parkrun must have one or two Event Directors who make sure events are delivered appropriately. They might have helped set up an event initially, and their duties include building relationships with landowners and liaising with parkrun HQ on any issues. Those in this role often work behind the scenes during the week updating risk assessments and ensuring volunteers are in place for the next week. They don't need to physically attend on a Saturday morning, when the Run Director will be in charge. However, many often do go along and often double as the Run Director or take on another volunteer role.

Run Director: The responsibility of ensuring a parkrun takes place safely on the day falls on the Run Director. They lead and support the team of volunteers and oversee the event from start to finish. They must decide whether to cancel a run due to adverse weather such as snow, or adjust a route if there are obstacles such as fallen trees following a gale. Their duties may begin in the week before the event by ensuring they have a team of volunteers in place and keeping an eye on the weather forecast. On the day, they arrive before 9am to oversee the course set-up and ensure the route is safe to run on. Before the run starts, they give the pre-run briefing which involves welcoming everyone, reminding them of the parkrun

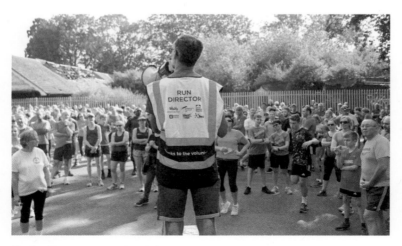

The Run Director oversees the whole event

DID YOU KNOW?

parkruns have gone ahead with Run Directors as young as ten, but under 18s must be accompanied throughout by an adult RD.

code, and giving any extra safety notices. At this point they mention any milestones happening that day, give a shout out to tourists, and ask everyone to give their thanks to the volunteers. Once they have started the runners off, the Run Director can't join in themselves as they must stay near the finish area in case there are any problems. They also shouldn't undertake any other volunteer roles so they are available to speak to any parkrunners who need their assistance, or respond to any emergency situations. Nick Oakley is one of the RDs at Colchester Castle parkrun in Essex. 'I enjoy it because it's a "communal enabling" role,' he says. 'When I was younger I played cricket, and that was only possible because of adults who organised it all. As an adult, I remember that and want to give back via parkrun, thus enabling community participation. I do it because it makes me feel good inside, and I never feel I need thanking.' Edric Hobbs, who has more than 344 volunteer credits to his name, agrees. 'Being RD at Shepton Mallet parkrun in Somerset is my favourite role. I like getting to the park nice and early and the buzz as the volunteers turn up. I enjoy giving the run briefing to our regulars and tourists and then it's nice to check the times on each of our laps and see how folk are doing. I'm immensely proud of our small event which I helped set up seven years ago.' Edric, 60, said skills needed to be RD include 'having the confidence to liaise with people from all walks of life. You need to know and believe in the ethos of parkrun, and being confident public speaking helps. You mustn't be afraid to enforce the few rules we have with some diplomacy.'

First Timers' Welcome: This role is essential because parkrun wants to ensure all those coming for the first time feel welcome and know what to expect from the event, and the route. The volunteer taking on this role will encourage all first timers to gather around them near the

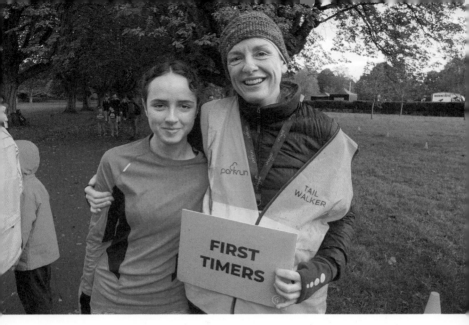

A volunteer at Florence Park in Oxford giving the First Timers Welcome before Tail Walking

start shortly before the race director's pre-run briefing. They will give a quick rundown of how parkrun works, and give the first timers an opportunity to ask any questions. Jen Whittle says she loves taking on this role because 'I get to chat to newcomers and be a friendly face'. It's also a favourite with Julia Fitzpatrick 'as I get to meet all of the tourists, tell them about our wonderful course in Andover and I can also run myself.' She adds: 'I really enjoy volunteering as it enables me to meet so many different people and adds another dimension to my parkrun, apart from just taking part. Volunteering is equally as rewarding.' Lana Donnison, a regular volunteer at Millennium Country parkrun in Bedfordshire, says the first timers' welcome is a great way 'to build up my confidence of speaking to a group of people.'

Event Day Course Check: The ideal job for an early riser. This person must walk, run or cycle the course on the morning of the event before the participants arrive to check it is safe for both runners and marshals, and free of obstacles. Those clocking up milestones often enjoy taking this role, as it means they can get a volunteer credit and then join in the run afterwards.

Timekeeper(s): An all-important role because gaining a finishing time for a parkrun is a key part of why many people do it, harking back to when it was started as a time trial. Timekeepers record the finish times of all participants using the parkrun volunteer app they must download (for free) on their phone prior to the event. So while participants mustn't forget their barcodes, timekeepers mustn't forget their mobiles, and ensure they are fully charged before leaving. Time-keepers use a stopwatch within the app which they must start when the run begins. They should keep their mobiles in flight mode while timing, to ensure there isn't a disruption from an incoming message or call. Then as each participant crosses the line, they tap their phone screen to log each finishing time. After the Tail Walker has been recorded as the final finisher, the results can be uploaded via the app to parkrun's results processing system. While parkruns can cope with just one timekeeper, having more than one is encouraged so there is a back-up in case technology fails on one device. Mike Tivnen says timekeeping is his favourite volunteer role, even though it can feel 'tense', especially at his home event, Bushy parkrun, where multiple people can finish at the same time. He says: 'I like the responsibility of timekeeping, it feels like an important job. It can be difficult to keep track of everyone finishing and it can go wrong. Once, I acciden-tally started the stopwatch too soon. But normally any issues can be resolved, especially when there is a second timekeeper.'

Finish Tokens: parkrun finish tokens are handed out not just so people can see what position they finished in, but so their position can be linked to their time. A volunteer will hand out the tokens in the finish funnel to each participant. An additional person can be assigned as 'finish token support' if enough volunteers are available. They will help hold and hand the tokens to the other volunteer. This is particu-larly useful at parkruns with a large number of participants to ensure people can keep flowing through the finish funnel. If they become too backed up, incoming runners and walkers won't be able to cross the line. Beatrice Merrigan said handing out the tokens at Black

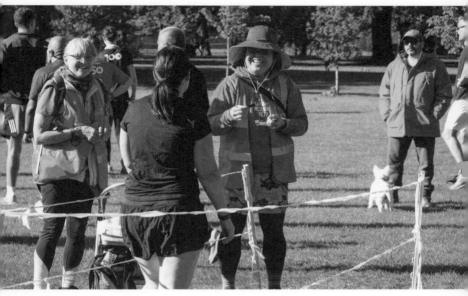

Handing out tokens at Cassiobury parkrun in Watford, Hertfordshire

Park parkrun, Buckinghamshire, where she volunteers regularly, is one of her favourite roles because 'it's fast paced and good fun, working closely with as a team to make it work. It is a big responsibility not to drop a token when we have over 500 people coming in quickly.' Linda Curley also loves doing this role at Wycombe Rye parkrun, Buckinghamshire, 'as you get a chance to say "well done" to everyone as they finish.' Ruth Cowlin agrees. She says: 'Giving out the finish tokens is really good because you see everyone and have a chance to say "congratulations". After volunteering I feel that I've contributed to a great community event and made everyone's Saturday start in a lovely way.'

Barcode Scanner(s): This role involves using the parkrun volunteer app again, and is needed so all participants can receive their results. The volunteer will scan the personal barcode of the finisher

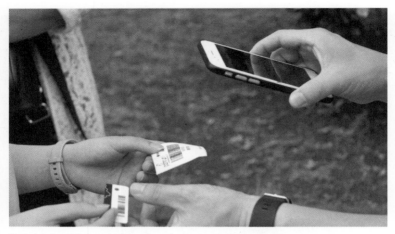

Scanning the all-important barcode and token at the finish

and the barcode on their finish token. They will then collect the finish token so it can be reused the following week. Jack Matthews, who volunteers and runs at Hastings parkrun in East Sussex, says 'I love barcode scanning because you get to talk to people when they finish and see how happy it makes them that they've got up and done parkrun.' Jack points out that if a venue is struggling for help, this is one of the roles you can combine with running and then volunteering. Stephanie Jordan agrees that barcode scanning is an excellent way to get to know people. 'At our small parkrun in Unisee, Germany, barcode scanning is quite a relaxed job and gives you the chance to chat to everyone, and learn their names.'

Tail Walker(s): This role is compulsory to maintain the parkrun rule that no-one ever finishes last. It also ensures the safety of everyone at the back of the field so no parkrunner who is struggling is left behind. Tail walking makes a great role for anyone who wants some exercise without running, and is popular with those who want to volunteer with their dogs. While one tail walker is essential, more are encouraged to create some camaraderie at the back of the field, and make the event more sociable for walkers. Tail walkers must

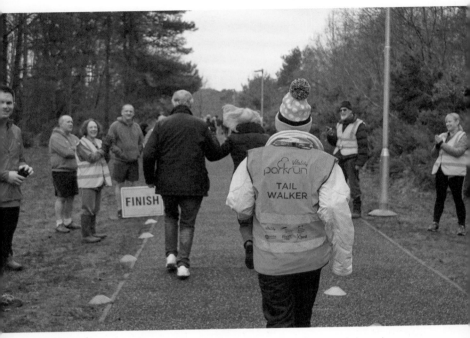

Tail walking is a good role for anyone who wants to exercise without running — and ensures that no one finishes last

be registered as parkrunners and have their personal barcode and a finish token scanned at the finish so they appear in the results. Louisa Harpham-Sou says she enjoys being a tail walker at Heaton Park, Manchester. 'I love to encourage people and hopefully they try to go a little faster than they would have without my encouragement,' she says. Elizabeth Ayres is another fan of Tail Walking. 'Walking around with the little legs, broken legs, old legs, and "just don't feel like running" legs, I get to hear so many life stories and why people are at parkrun,' she enthuses. 'I love it and for those who are struggling, they get me as their own personal cheerleader.'

The following volunteer roles aren't deemed compulsory by parkrun HQ, but filling them is encouraged to enhance the smooth running of the event:

Marshals: These volunteers direct and encourage participants around the course with enthusiasm. They need to be positioned at key points where a runner might take a wrong turn, or where they need to give a warning over any hazards such as tree roots or tight corners. They might need to remind runners to keep to one side of the course on a lapped, or out and back route, to avoid collisions. Some courses will need more marshals than others depending on the route. Many around the world which have few participants and volunteers manage with no marshals at all and use signs and cones to direct people. At junior parkruns, however, marshals are compulsory to ensure no children go off in the wrong direction, as often the older ones will be running without a parent or guardian. Anne Kelly, 48, from Manchester says marshalling at junior parkrun is a really rewarding role: 'There's nothing better than hearing a junior parkrunner shout "thank you marshal"! Or giving you a high five as they go past.'

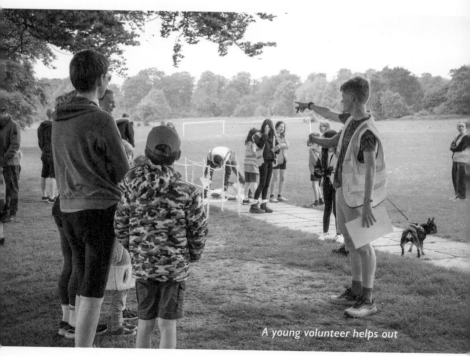

A young volunteer helps out

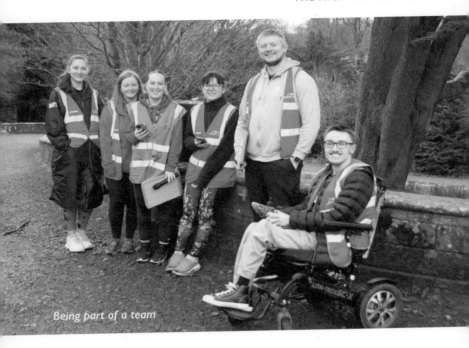

Being part of a team

Pre-event Setup and Post-event Close Down: Does what it says on the tin – the pre-event volunteers help set up the course by for example, putting up k/mile markers or directional signs, laying out cones to show people where to go, and erecting a finish funnel. These will all then be removed afterwards by the Post-Event Close Down team/volunteer who will ensure the area where the run has taken place is left as it was found with no signs, litter, or kit left behind. Some parkruns might assign an additional 'Equipment Storage and Deliver' volunteer to look after all the event equipment in between events, and bring them along again each Saturday. Jamie Moore, who volunteers at Sittingbourne, says the pre-course set-up is another opportunity to combine volunteering with taking part as a runner, and get to know the route before you run it.

Volunteer Coordinator: Each parkrun event page has a volunteer roster showing who has signed up for the roles in the forthcoming weeks. The co-ordinator keeps this roster up-to-date and ensures there are enough helpers each week for the run to go ahead. They'll have to check emails coming in from volunteers and appeal on social media channels for help if they are short on any roles. This is a role that can be done without having to attend the actual event. If there isn't a volunteer coordinator available, often the Run Director for that week's event might take on this role.

Funnel Managers: These volunteers encourage finishers to move through the finish funnel whilst staying in the order they crossed the line. This prevents bunching at the line as more people finish, and ensures the published results are accurate. At parkruns with high attendances, dual funnels are often set up to ensure the flow of finishers which requires teamwork and communication between the funnel manager, number checker and those giving out the finishing tokens to ensure finishing positions don't get mixed up. At junior parkruns, the funnel manager is another compulsory role as the children are more likely to move out of order, or leave the funnel before getting their token.

Number Checker: This role is particularly useful at large events where lots of people might be crossing the line at a similar time, and then have to queue along the finish funnel to get their token. The number checker will note what position someone was in when they crossed the line, eg, 44th, and then check that when they reach the volunteer giving out the tokens, they are given number 44. If there is a discrepancy they will have to make a note and help resolve it before the results are published. If there aren't enough volunteers, this role could be combined with being the Funnel Manager.

Results Processor: Once the timekeeper has finished recording the results, this volunteer can help check for any mistakes before it is sent to parkrun's database to be published. Errors might occur if someone has ducked out of the funnel or their barcode didn't scan. The result processor can liaise with the RD, Funnel Manager and Number Checker to see if they made a note of any potential problems so they can be resolved. If short on volunteers, this is a job the timekeeper could also do.

Token Sorting Volunteer: This person is responsible for collecting all the tokens at the end of the event and putting them back in numerical order for the following week. Some will take the tokens home to do this. Others do it in a cafe after an event with the help of the others to share the work and make it more sociable.

Volunteers to Support Those with Disabilities: The 'Sign Language Support' role can be taken by anyone who is able to sign the First Timer's welcome the pre-run briefing for the benefit of those who are deaf or and hard of hearing. Volunteer 'VI Guides' are also welcomed to assist visually impaired participants around a course. For anyone who needs a guide runner and doesn't already know someone they can take with them to parkrun, the RD is the best point of contact to arrange one. There's a vacancy on the volunteer roster each week, and if it hasn't been filled the week a visually impaired participant is due to attend, the RD can contact a parkrun regular to see if they can step in. This is how Clare Mortimer first became a guide runner at Southwark parkrun in London. Clare knew the route well having done it nearly 200 times since 2017 along with her daughter so she was asked by the RD if she could help a blind runner who was attending one day. 'I guess the RD knew that I was very familiar with the course and I was used to running with kids, so I wasn't afraid of the responsibility,' Clare recalls. Clare has since been a Guide Runner 16 times and finds it really rewarding. 'I'm a huge believer that parkrun can be accessible to everyone. Guiding allows me to be part of making that true for anyone who is visually impaired,' she says. 'When we're running most of the runners are really considerate and supportive so it is a great reminder of the community side of parkrun. And you get both running and volunteering credits, so it's a super role!' To be a good Guide Runner, Clare says: 'You definitely need to be thinking/watching one step ahead – being a Mum is great training for this, all those outings predicting where a toddler on a scooter would go next is probably where I learned this one! You have to be a clear communicator so instructions can be heard, and know your left from your right! It helps if you enjoy a chat so that you build trust with the runner you're guiding.'

Parkwalker: This is a separate, non-compulsory role to being the Tail Walker. These volunteers should walk slightly ahead of the Tail Walker at a typical walking speed 'to demonstrate that walking is welcome at parkrun'. This role was introduced as part of the 'park-walk at parkrun' campaign launched in 2018 to encourage more people to feel at home by walking the entire 5k.

Pacers: Some parkruns have regular weeks where volunteers run at a certain pace to accompany people on their walk/run, or to help them achieve a finishing time they have been striving for. The pacers usually wear blue bibs with the number of the finishing time they are aiming to cross the line in on their back. Kelly Curran says she loves doing this role at Cranbrook Country Park parkrun in Devon because: 'I get so much good feedback from people who run around me.' She says: 'People have said they have come to our particular parkrun because of the presence of pacers who help and encourage them. It gives me all the warm fuzzies knowing I have actively been a part of helping someone achieve their goal.' Richard Sved, a dedicated volunteer who has surpassed the 400 milestone in various roles at St Albans parkrun, Hertfordshire, says: 'More recently I've taken up being a pacer and I enjoy it tremendously. I love the challenge of hitting a specific time and the fact that I have a posse of people behind me who are thrilled to be helped to the time they wanted to get.' John Broom, who has attended nearly 600 parkruns, is another

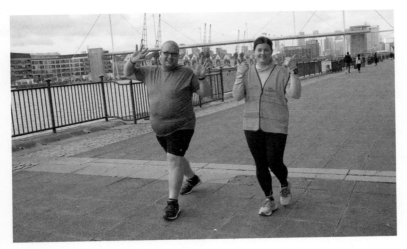

Enjoying a walk at Victoria Dock parkrun, London

who has found pacing to be a fulfilling role as 'it involves physical effort and pace judgement, whilst giving an immediately tangible boost to anyone you pace to a PB.'

Photographers and Report Writers: These roles help create more of a buzz around parkrun and allow people to see and read about the events. Photographers can take photos and videos of participants, but these must only be shared on the parkrun pages. Bruce Bryan, a regular at Elliott Heads Beach parkrun in Queensland, Australia, says: 'My favourite role is photographer, because I am able to capture the joy participants get from parkrun, as well as showcasing the beautiful surroundings of our local events.' Lee-Anne Brakeswood agrees being a photographer is rewarding as 'it is about keeping memories alive'. Graham Smith, who has volunteered as a photographer at parkruns in Bedfordshire, Buckinghamshire and Hertfordshire, adds: 'The photographer role gives me a chance to volunteer at the same time as doing something I enjoy. I really feel part of the event, especially with all the waves and smiles. Hopefully the parkrunners enjoy seeing their photos afterwards too.' Meanwhile, the report writer can share as much or as little information as they like on that week's event. They usually cover who the volunteers were, and anything notable such as milestones, the weather, or people taking part for a special reason eg on their hen do. Some people submit a report after visiting a venue as a tourist to share their experience. The report will only be published on the event and social media pages of the parkrun being written about.

Car Park Marshal: parkrun encourages people to walk, run or use public transport to get to their events. For those who have to drive, a volunteer might be on hand to show them the best places to park safely and sensibly.

Warm-up coordinator: This role is only compulsory at junior parkruns to increase the enjoyment of young participants and get them ready to run. The volunteer will lead them through a series of moves on the spot such as arm swings and star jumps. Vicki Skip says: 'I love being a warm up leader at junior parkrun. I just trained as a personal trainer so it has helped my confidence getting the group motivated and ready to go.' Benjamin Weaver, who is a co-event director at Burslem Park junior parkrun in Stoke-on-Trent, adores getting everyone moving and smiling. 'I love being Warm Up Leader – especially star jumping in a circle. I love seeing families and friends all warming up and then running/walking together and the park

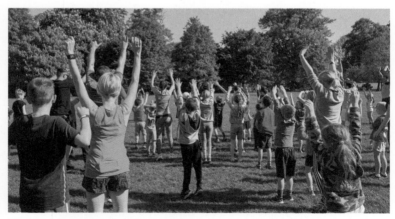

Hands up who wants to do junior parkrun?

being full of life. We even kept our warm ups going live on our Facebook page during lockdown when events were cancelled,' he says. 'It's lovely that we've built a wonderful volunteering community, made up of a wide range of people from all walks of life. Then we pack away and it's like we were never there. It's great to see juniors getting involved in volunteering too.'

DID YOU KNOW?

Nicki Clark, who is in her fifties, became the first ever parkrunner to reach the 1,000 volunteer milestone in March 2024.

AMBASSADOR ROLES

As parkrun grew, more volunteers were needed to work behind the scenes, taking on roles that fell outside the remit of being present on a Saturday (or Sunday mornings for junior parkruns) morning. So in 2013, the ambassador scheme was created. Those passionate about parkrun can apply for this unpaid role, and then they might be matched to a job dependent on their skills. For example, someone who is an expert at IT might help manage the parkrun system when all the results are coming in from various events on a Saturday morning, while someone with calm people skills might cover the critical incident line each weekend. Other ambassadors might help a new parkrun get started by supporting the newly formed event team as an event support ambassador, a job Edric Hobbs has undertaken as well as being an RD. Explaining his duties, he says: 'I help new teams start events and do the paperwork. An event support ambassador looks after six events, helping them to run smoothly and advising events on any rule changes. We are a face-to-face link between the event core team and head office.' parkrun describes its ambassadors as 'the guardians, advocates, protectors and champions of parkrun'. At the start of 2024 parkrun had 750 ambassadors globally, with 350 of those in the UK, undertaking a wide range of duties. Conferences are often held where they can meet one another and learn more about parkrun.

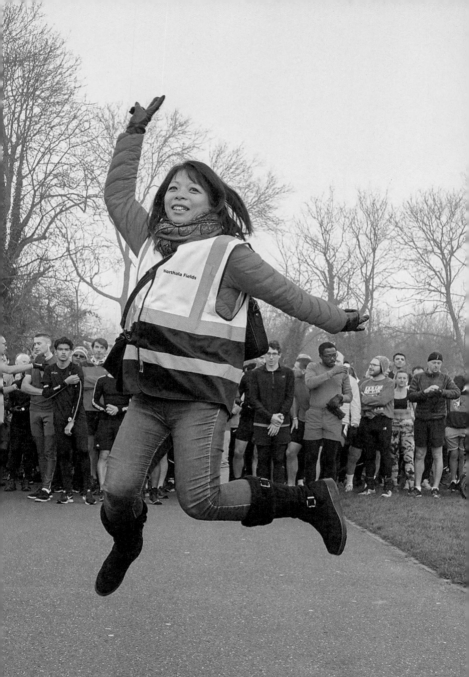

Leaping into action: a run director

CHAPTER FOUR:

A DAY IN THE LIFE OF A PARKRUN

7.30am: It's a frosty Saturday morning at the end of February 2024 for event 581 of Colwick parkrun in Nottingham. Jonathan Shirt is the first volunteer to arrive to do the pre-course check. He sets off on his bike following the route through the picturesque country park, owned by Nottingham County Council. The course runs alongside the River Trent and then loops around two big lakes which are popular with wild swimmers and wildlife. The paths used to all be trails which often became boggy and slippery in the winter months. So much so, that one section was affectionately referred to as 'shoe-sucker straight' by parkrunners who struggled through the quagmire. But in 2023, the council concreted over all the paths, which now provide a fast, smooth surface which Jonathan whirls around, checking for obstacles such as fallen tree branches and ice patches, given that the temperature dropped below zero overnight. He finds the finishing line is totally submerged due to one of the lakes flooding in recent heavy rainfall. Luckily, the team has already prepared for this and can use a different path as an alternative finishing straight. As per parkrun guidance, this means the route will be very slightly longer than 5k. When alternative courses are used, it is recommended they are longer so people don't set inaccurate PBs on a course that might be shorter than 5k, and then be unable to break them again on the accurate course.

8am: Andrew meets with Run Director Helen near the course start and reports that while the grass surrounding the paths is frosty, the route itself is ice-free and is not slippery. It is ultimately the RD's decision whether to cancel an event and Helen agrees that given there is no ice on the path and the sun is already coming up to make temperatures warmer, they are good to go. Now he's done the pre-course check, Andrew will join in the parkrun, meaning he's been able to volunteer and run on the same day. He first started parkrunning with his Labrador, Diesel, and has since clocked up 220 runs and eight volunteer stints. He said: 'parkrun is Diesel's favourite day of the week but he's injured at the moment which is why I was able to do the pre-course check. I've also been a marshal before and done the token sorting. I enjoy getting to know people by volunteering. When I come down and run with Diesel, I might see the odd person I know and have a chat but I get to know a bigger group of people by volunteering, which is nice.'

On her way to meet Andrew, Helen and her husband and fellow volunteer, Frazer, have collected equipment including sign posts from a lock-up in the park. They carry this to their next meeting point with the other volunteers.

8.15am: The team of 32 volunteers meet near to where the finish will be set up. Helen welcomes everyone and assigns their roles, ensuring they all know what they are doing. She hands out lanyards with information on what to do in the event of an emergency, such as the passcode to access the defibrillators and mobile numbers of the RDs. There's time to chit chat, take pictures and catch up. Helen explains it is going to be a special event as it will be the 500th parkrun for regular attendee Karen Parkin. She has been going since the very first event in June 2011 and is the first person whose home parkrun is Colwick to reach this milestone. To celebrate, they have set up a table next to where the barcode scanners will stand so people can help themselves to some cakes brought along to mark the occasion. Helen adds it will be a poignant celebration as another regular, Paul Stacey, would also have reached the 500 milestone today but sadly died suddenly towards the end of the previous year. There are also cakes provided in his honour and his partner, Sarah Bull, will run round with Karen.

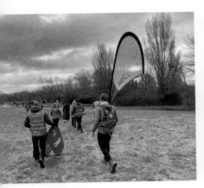

Colwick parkrun volunteers walk to the start

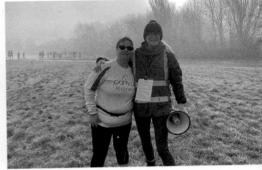

Karen Parkin on her 500th run with Run Director Helen

8.40am The marshals head out on the course to their positions. One of them is Morag Whitworth, 70. She only took up running when she was 64 but has already racked up more than 125 parkruns, including ones in Canada and Australia, and has volunteered 62 times. Speaking of volunteering, she said: 'I started doing it a lot more after I donated a kidney. At that time, I couldn't walk far or run at all so it was great to still be able to participate. I've got to know a lot more people from volunteering which is great. I can run again now so I do that or walk some weeks, sometimes with my son, daughter and grandchildren. I enjoy walking, running and volunteering – it's a great reason to get up on a Saturday morning and it keeps me fit.'

8.45am: Jason Randall, who is the funnel manager for the day, starts setting up the funnel using stakes and tape with the help of some of the other volunteers. He says: 'I adore parkrun, it's the best way to get my weekend going and it has helped me make some fantastic friends. I have done 238 parkruns at 88 different locations. There is a great sense of community and it brings everyone together.' Jason is volunteering today while he takes a rest from running due to a knee injury. It's his first time as funnel manager and he explains its importance: 'I have to help everyone get through the funnel in the right

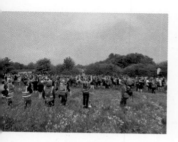

The race briefing

order and ensure they get the right token.' He predicts that at around 26 minutes (after the start) the finish line will get fraught for two or three minutes with the bulk of runners coming through in droves and multiple people crossing the line at the same time. 'So that will be a testing time!' he predicts.

8.50am: Helen and volunteers for the First Time briefing and timekeeping head to the start where parkrunners are already assembling along a path behind the start line. Some are waiting and chatting, others are doing final warm up jogs and dynamic stretches, while others are setting up their running playlists on their mobiles. Dogs who can't wait to get going bark excitedly over the hum of conversation.

8.55am: Volunteer Alison calls First Timers to join her at a flag near the start line for the first timers' briefing. Around a dozen attend. They are either taking part in parkrun for the very first time, are new to Colwick because they are tourists, or visiting because their usual parkrun in Nottingham has been cancelled by the wintry weather. Alison holds up a map of the course which she uses to explain the route and points out any potential hazards along the way. One key turning point is known as 'Roy's split' – named in memory of an elderly volunteer called Roy, who would marshal at that point most weeks until his death in 2020. Alison reassures everyone they won't get lost as there are plenty of marshals to direct them today and she wishes them well in their run/walk. Alison says she enjoys doing the first timers' briefing as it 'helps people feel welcome and included.' 'There's a lot to say and we are given guidance on this but you also have to keep it brief so you don't delay the start,' she explains. She enjoys 'giving back' as a volunteer. The role means she can also then take part, which she does today by joining the other parkrunners on the start line after finishing her briefing.

8.58am: Helen gives her briefing as RD via a megaphone reminding everyone of the parkrun code of conduct and sharing the news of milestones reached today, including Karen's 500th. She asks if there are any tourists and discovers visitors from Maidenhead and Redhill. She then leads a round of applause for all the volunteers.

9am: Helen shouts 'Go!' The parkrunners are off and the time-keepers start their stopwatches. Masses of parkrunners go past and Helen predicts today will be one of their highest turnouts. She hopes they have enough finish tokens. Helen first attended Colwick parkrun at event three 'and never left'. She has volunteered more than 760 times and is a regular RD at Rushcliffe junior parkrun in Nottingham too. 'I love the whole thing', she says. 'I love the community, seeing people coming back each week and hearing their stories. I love the little things I see each week like people who have never met before patting one another on the back in the finish funnel after pushing one another around, and then they know one another next time. Moments like that are priceless. I love being RD at junior parkrun as I get to see the children coming every week growing up.' Helen's husband, Frazer, acting as a timekeeper today, joined her at her first event and hundreds more since. He saw how captivated she was when she attended and she turned and told him, 'this will change our lives'. She was right. As well as volunteering most weeks at Colwick in various roles, they volunteer when they are in other parts of the country too. They both became ambassadors for a time, helping new events get set up. Then ten years ago, Helen became the Head of Event Delivery for parkrun UK so now works

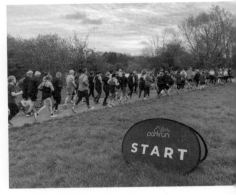

Colwick parkrun start

full-time for parkrun HQ. She admits there is nowhere she would rather be on a weekend morning. She loves volunteering more than running. 'If I run it, I'll look at the results after and see loads of people who were there who I didn't get to speak to. When I'm RD I'm like a butterfly fluttering around the finish. I get to see everyone, deal with any issues they have, and of course I'm on standby in case of any emergencies.'

9.05: Helen and the timekeepers head back to the finish line in time to see the parkrunners come by as they enter their first loop of the park. They cheer people on as they pass at various paces, some with dogs, some pushing running buggies, some running with children, some with guide runners. Then come the walkers, some elderly, some using walking poles, and some power-walking in pairs while they chat. The parkwalk volunteers pass and not long after that a group of Tail Walkers.

9.17: Shortly after the Tail Walkers have passed the first finisher comes in – Joshua Smith, a teenager who runs for Notts AC – with a time of 17.07. More club runners follow, with the field still quite spread out with about five to 10 seconds between each finisher. The first female – Beatrix Perks – crosses the line in 21.47 and then the flow of runners keeps increasing, with finishers every few seconds. Frazer and fellow timekeeper, Sophie, a teenager who is volunteering as part of her Duke of Edinburgh Award, are on either side of the finish funnel tapping their mobiles each time a runner goes over the line. This records their time while the stopwatch keeps running. Timekeeping is a lot easier now that timers can use

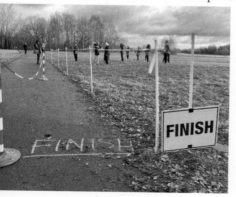

Colwick parkrun finish funnel

the parkrun app on their own mobile phones, as previously they had to use stopwatches linked to laptops. It can be tiring standing in place for up to an hour, so Frazer has brought his own camping chair to sit on. Arry Nathan, a Colwick parkrun regular, finishes in 24.37. He has run more than 200 of his 417 parkruns at Colwick since 2012, as well as regularly volunteering. Arry, 50, a consultant anaesthetist and sub-3 hour marathon runner, says 'I'm a parkrun addict and include parkrun as part of my marathon training. But I actually love volunteering more than running – I've done all roles, including Run Directing here 64 times. The community is the best thing about Colwick. People are kind, friendly and welcoming, making others feel at home.'

9.25am: Frazer and Sophie have their work cut out tapping continuously as the runners start coming in thick and fast. Sam Algar, a sprightly teenager volunteering as number checker, covers many steps dashing back and forth between the finish line and the end of the funnel where the tokens are being handed out to ensure everyone is getting the correct finish position token. He said he loves being involved as parkrun is 'a nice place to be, even when it is tipping it down as people seem to be even more friendly then.' Thankfully the weather has stayed dry today and the sun has come out.

9.26am: Runners with dogs, runners pushing buggies, friends running together, people sprinting one another to the line all start flowing in thick and fast as Jason predicted. 'I ran the whole way!' one finisher exclaims to her friends who are cheering for her on the sidelines. Others shake hands in the funnel and congratulate one another. 'You kept me going there,' one man says to another, who he finished just behind. With the runners streaming in now, it soon becomes quite congested and the volunteers handing out the finishing tokens have to work at speed to keep everyone moving. A bottleneck means the finishers start getting backed-up over the line, which could prevent others coming in from finishing in an accurate time. So, Tony, a parkrun regular who has finished running, offers to help out and Helen throws him a marshal bib to wear. Along with Jason, he instructs everyone to keep moving along the funnel and to stay in their finishing position while Sam keeps running up and down to make sure the finishing positions remain correct. Once leaving the funnel, the parkrunners head over to a grassy area beside the finish to wait in line to have their barcodes scanned. Many then hang around to chat, take selfies, cheer the other runners over the line, or grab one of the milestone cakes.

9.36: Karen crosses the line for her 500th time with a huge smile on her face, holding hands with Sarah. It's a bittersweet moment for Sarah running her 165th parkrun in memory of Paul.

9.43: Joggers and walkers varying in ages from under 10 to over 80 continue to finish. Helen is certain it will be one of their highest turnouts ever.

10am: The tail walker crosses the line and takes their finish token – 500! Colwick's second highest ever (the record is 573 on New Year's Day 2019). A completely apt number to celebrate Karen and Paul's 500ths. 'What were the odds on that!' Helen exclaims. Sam, Jason and other volunteers start taking down the finishing funnel while Helen starts packing up the remaining cakes and takes down the camp table they were set up on. Many of the finishers have headed to a cafe 100m away and some of the volunteers will join them there. Frazer explains they always used to all go to the cafe to process the results but thanks to the app, he can now do it all at the finish line if he wants to. This is how he will do it today and he first checks the results over with Helen. A couple of people's personal barcodes wouldn't scan, so Helen took down their barcode numbers and they are now manually uploaded into the results. Frazer then finds there's an issue that is preventing the results being uploaded to the parkrun server. The number of tokens handed out does not

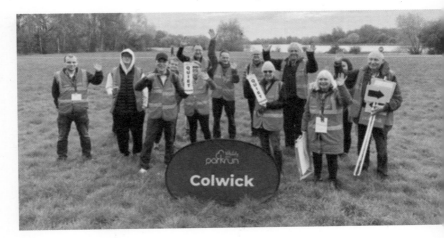

Volunteers at Colwick parkrun

match the number of finishing times recorded. After a quick chat with the finishing token team, they discover two tokens must have stuck together and been handed out to cause the anomaly. With this resolved, Frazer can now upload the results to parkrun's main system. Just a few minutes later, all the participants will be pinged an email with their individual result from the morning.

10.25am: Helen thanks and says goodbye to the remaining volunteers. She and Frazer carry the equipment back to their car. Some of it they will leave in the lock-up in the park, and the rest they will take home with them to pass on to next week's RDs. The park is busy now with dog walkers and families out for walks with children on bikes and scooters. No trace of the parkrun has been left behind. It is like it has never been there. But 532 people go home with a spring in their step after spending the morning with their parkrun family. 'Same again next week!' Helen says happily as she heads home to post photos of the event on the Colwick parkrun Facebook page and write up the run report.

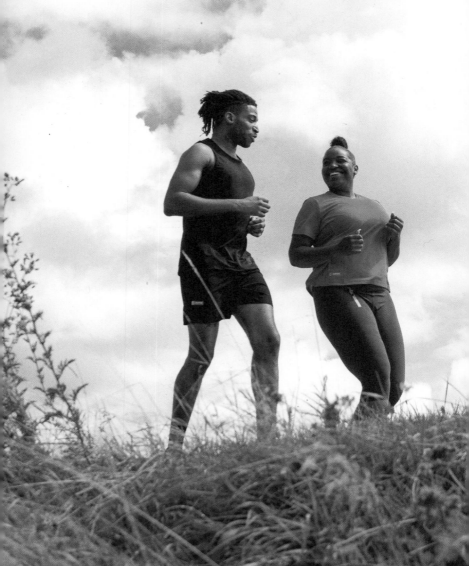

The health benefits of parkrun are clear. Photo: Contra Movement-169

CHAPTER FIVE

WHY YOU SHOULD PARKRUN FOR YOUR HEALTH AND WELL-BEING

PHYSICAL HEALTH BENEFITS

The World Health Organisation (WHO) recommends adults do at least 150–300 minutes of moderate to intense aerobic physical activity per week. It has made these recommendations based on numerous studies on the impact of exercise that have found it has 'significant health benefits for hearts, bodies and minds'. Running in particular has been found to be an excellent way to meet physical activity needs. To name just a few examples of the benefits – it strengthens bones, lowers blood pressure, eases anxiety and depression and helps maintain a healthy body weight. It contributes to the prevention and management of a huge range of diseases such as heart failure, diabetes and some cancers. Exercise also helps you live longer. The WHO states that people who are 'insufficiently active have a 20-30 per cent increased risk of death compared to people who are sufficiently active'. This is backed up by a recent study in the International Journal of Environmental Research and Public Health, which found that 75 minutes of jogging a week – versus none at all – boosted life span by approximately 12 years. If you attend a

DID YOU KNOW?

Globally, one in four adults do not meet the global recommended levels of physical activity.

parkrun once a week you can do a big chunk of this exercise in a single morning. If you are unable to run, walking is also an excellent way to keep fit, especially if you can do it at a brisk pace. It will help you build stamina, burn calories and strengthen your muscles. So, if you can walk or run at parkrun, you will be boosting your health and wellbeing. This has been proven by a team of academics from the University of Sydney, led by Associate Professor Dr Anne Grunseit, who reviewed research carried out between 2004-19 on the health and wellbeing of parkrunners in the UK and Australia. parkrun participants showed improvements in fitness, total physical activity and mood. Anne, who regularly parkruns herself, said: 'Most encouraging is that the positive effects were largest for those who were less active when they registered with parkrun, and that there is a dose response – the more frequently someone participates in parkrun events, the bigger the positive impact.'

She added: 'According to the research we reviewed, parkrun's appeal seems to come from the sense of achievement, physical move-ment, being in pleasant surroundings and the opportunity for social interaction. The volunteering aspect of parkrun gives people the

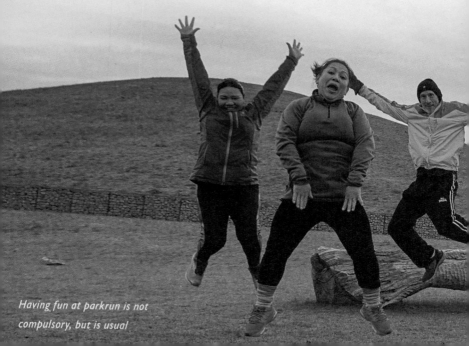

Having fun at parkrun is not compulsory, but is usual

opportunity to participate even if they do not run or walk the 5k. parkrun also gives people who do not normally think of themselves as runners a new and unifying identity – that of being a parkrunner – which connects them to a community based around being active.'

MENTAL HEALTH BENEFITS

When it comes to mental health, a recent study carried out by the University of South Australia concluded that exercise is such a powerful tool in enhancing our well-being, it should be 'a mainstay approach' in the management of depression, anxiety and mental health disorders. The comprehensive research involved 128,119 participants. It found that 'physical activity is 1.5 times more effective than counselling or the leading medications'. parkrun founder Paul Sinton-Hewitt has been vocal himself about how running has boosted his mental health throughout his life. Numerous studies have found that exercise can enhance mentally well being because it prompts our brains to release feel-good hormones such as endorphins. These hormones boost happiness and self-esteem and improve the quality of

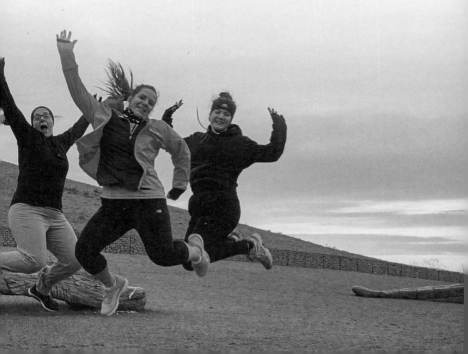

our sleep. Many have felt this 'runner's high' after a parkrun.

A public health dissertation published by Orla Siobhan Purdon in 2021 reported that parkrun isn't just a mood-lifter for those who joined in by being physically active. Positive mental health outcomes were also reported by those who attended as volunteers, because it has made them feel connected to others. On top of this, just being outside experiencing the restorative effects of nature at a parkrun can have immense benefits. Numerous studies have found that proximity to green space and being in an outdoor, natural environment is associated with lower stress levels, and can improve symptoms of depression and anxiety.

'PARKRUN SAVED US'

Dawn Barsby, 54, from Leicester, experienced first-hand how parkrun can boost mental health.

She recalls: 'I had a mental health breakdown in November 2021 and couldn't leave the house or be around people for months (parkrun hadn't been running for a lot of this time because of Covid). When I felt better, I decided to do some parkrun tourism. This tourism gave me a different reason to attend rather than running. It was about going somewhere different and seeing the different routes.' In the summer of 2022, Dawn did Faskally Forest parkrun in Perthshire, Scotland, in the morning and then broke her ankle on Cairngorm Mountain in the afternoon. 'This is where my parkrun journey completely changed', Dawn says. 'My ankle break was a bad one which required surgery and metal work. I was stuck in the house, not able to go out or do anything. I knew this wasn't good for my mental health. I emailed my home parkrun – Braunstone parkrun in Leicester – and asked if there was anything I could do while being immobile. I was given the task of token sorting so I attended on my knee scooter. Once I could manage on crutches, I started to barcode scan, and I would take my chair to sit on as much as possible. I loved chatting to the other volunteers while waiting for the first finishers and congratulating everyone as I scanned their barcode.'

Dawn, who now works as an apprentice skills coach, has racked up more than 100 parkruns and volunteered more than 55 times.

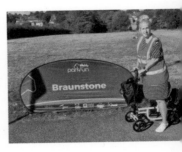

Dawn Barsby volunteering after breaking her ankle

'Doctors have told me not to run again as I have permanent damage in my ankle but parkrun is still very much a part of my life. If I'm not volunteering, I join in by walking instead – something I'd never considered before breaking my ankle as I thought you were supposed to run it,' she said. 'I can definitely say parkrun has saved me. It stopped me from getting into a dark place and having another breakdown. Now I enjoy walking and talking and then going for a coffee with friends after. It's a highlight of my week.'

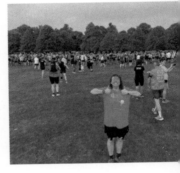

Celia Stanworth at Bushy parkrun

Celia Stanworth, a 39-year-old science teacher, says she might not be here if it wasn't for parkrun as it helped her following the tragic loss of her baby.

'parkrun has saved my life,' she says. 'It gave me a sense of purpose, targets, a group of friends, and something to look forward to after my baby, Eliza, was stillborn. At this time, I struggled with thoughts of suicide and self harm.' Celia wanted to do something to be healthy so she started with a Couch to 5k plan with the aim of completing a parkrun. This helped her channel her thoughts towards achieving a goal after a tough summer. 'My friends knew that parkrun would be something I loved as I'm autistic and like collecting things, and they agreed to come with me,' she said. 'I completed my first few at Watermeadows parkrun in Towcester by doing a combination of walking and jogging. The volunteers were always so welcoming and supportive. I still remember telling the final marshal on the route that I had run the whole thing and her face was pure joy at my achievement. I went on to have another baby and I ran pregnant with him for as long as possible before switching to walking.' Celia has now completed 107 parkruns and gained 50 volunteer credits, while eldest daughter, aged four, has done a couple of junior parkruns. Celia says: 'The impact parkrun has had on my mental health has been significant and it has massively helped my physical health too, as well as my social life.'

Meanwhile, Joe Spraggins, 34, from Dorking, Surrey, has also found parkrun a saviour for his mental health during an ongoing struggle with long-term illness. Joe was already a runner when he first heard about parkrun in 2014 and he started attending with his wife, Katie, to meet up with their running friends and see how fast he could go. Then in 2021, everything changed. After becoming unwell, Joe went from doing epic endurance challenges like Ironman Triathlons to not even having the energy to get out of bed.

'For someone who loves being active and outdoors, this was very hard to take. I didn't recognise myself anymore. For the first few months when I was unwell, I wasn't really able to leave the house. I could barely move and I couldn't find any joy anywhere. I missed my old life and seeing all my running buddies,' Joe recalls.

When his fatigue and sickness slightly eased, Joe, a senior finance manager at the Gym Group, decided to make attending his local parkrun/junior parkrun in Surrey his one outing of the week. 'I wasn't going to let my illness take this away from me. If I wasn't well enough to walk, I could volunteer,' he says. Doctors still haven't got to the bottom of Joe's condition, suggesting it could be long Covid, Chronic fatigue (ME) or another enduring post-viral fatigue.

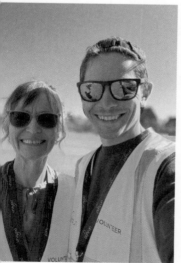

Joe Spraggins volunteering with his mum Melanie

Throughout his struggles, parkrun has remained a constant, and Joe is now approaching his 200th volunteer credit, including being RD at Reigate Priory junior parkrun a number of times. 'Going to parkrun every week has given me back a small sense of achievement and purpose, as well as additional support from friends and family who I see on a weekend morning. It gives me something to look forward to during week days when I feel really poorly and struggle to see the point in anything. Being outside in the fresh air with others has kept me going and allowed me to keep a bit of sanity and peace,' he says.

PARKRUN ON PRESCRIPTION

parkrun is well aware of how exercise can enhance physical and mental health, which is why it is so keen to get as many people as possible at its events. In 2018, it started the 'parkrun practice initiative' in the UK, Australia and Ireland, in collaboration with the Royal College of General Practitioners (RCGP). This project encourages GP practices to develop close links with their local parkrun event(s) and encourage staff and patients to join in for the many health benefits. At the time of publication, more than 1,800 GP practices around the UK had signed up. Dr Abbie Brooks, a GP partner at Priory Medical Group, is a big fan of the project. She told RCGP's research into the benefits of the parkrun practice initiative: 'I often recommend parkrun to my patients as it has been such a big part of my own journey with movement and exercise. parkrun is so much more than a run, it is the social element and community that can really benefit many of my patients. I love being able to talk about parkrun in my consultations.'

PARKRUN VERSUS CANCER

Not only has exercise been found to reduce the risk of getting cancer, it can provide big benefits for those who have been diagnosed. This is because it can help reduce fatigue, improve fitness and mental well-being and boost the immune system. Research is being carried out looking into how it may also reduce the side effects of chemotherapy, reduce the risk of cancer recurring and prolong survival. Macmillan Cancer Support is one of parkrun's official charity partners. It encourages people to join in parkrun for their health and wellbeing, while parkrun promotes the charity's services to make people more aware of the support they can receive if they or a loved one has cancer. Another charity called MOVE Charity also advocates exercise for those with cancer. At numerous parkruns across the UK, it has '5kYourWay' groups who attend on the last Saturday of every month. Each group is led by a 5kYourWay ambassador, whose life has been touched by cancer. While the charity encourages people with cancer to attend parkrun every week, the monthly meet ups offer extra support and the chance to meet other people in a similar situation. Sarah Mawhinney, 60, is one of the people who has experienced the positive power of parkrun thanks to 5kYourWay. She has taken part in 160 parkruns, the majority of which were after she was diagnosed with breast cancer in 2019. 'My diagnosis after a routine mammogram came as a total shock, at the time I was really fit, regularly competing in Ironman triathlons and I'd just run the London Marathon,' she recalled. 'I would need surgery, chemotherapy, radiotherapy and hormone treatment. I knew staying active would help me to cope with this, and that exercise may help reduce the risk of recurrence, so I started attending my local parkrun in Shropshire regularly. It helped me so much both mentally and physically.' Sarah knew others could benefit too, so she set up a 5kYourWay group at Shrewsbury parkrun in 2021. 'I love seeing how it helps others who have had their lives affected by cancer. Coming together for a walk or run and chat over coffee afterwards can be so supportive,' she enthuses. 'I always stress to people who are reluctant to join in that it is not about running. We have members who would never have contemplated going to parkrun before their diagnosis.'

Allyson Kent, 59, is one of the people who would never have considered parkrunning prior to her diagnosis of breast and then ovarian cancer when she was 55-years-old. 'I have never been a runner and I never imagined I would be,' she recalls. 'After my diagnosis, I wanted to do all I could so my body could be the best it could be for the treatment ahead. So, when I heard about 5kYourWay, it sounded like a great opportunity to get active.' Allyson set up a group at Beverley Westwood parkrun in East Yorkshire, and is now proud to say she has done more than 73 parkruns, sometimes attending following treatment such as platelet infusions and blood transfusions. 'I love love love parkrun,' she says. 'I never imagined I would be a runner and now I'm doing parkruns when on holiday in the UK and on Christmas Day. parkrun has helped me so much. I'm now the fittest I have ever been. I hope I can inspire others to have a go.'

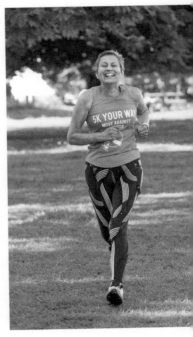

Allyson Kent, 5kYourWay Ambassador

COMMUNITY IMPACT

parkrun is a community in itself that people become part of as soon as they register. In locations where parkrun events exist, they also create their own sense of community for those who attend. While every parkrun follows the same format and ethos, there will still be individual differences in the events based on regular attendees, quirks of the course and the demographic of the surrounding population. Some parkruns love having a 'PB bell' at the finish people can ring after running a fastest time, some might have a marshal who never misses a week and everyone knows the spot they will be cheering on. Others provide music for the passing participants on special occasions, such as St Albans parkrun in Hertfordshire, who have their own brass bands made up of parkrunners, and Cyclopark parkrun in Kent, and Dewsbury parkrun in West Yorkshire, who have choirs. At Waterworks parkrun in Belfast, Northern Ireland, they have an RD famed for singing the run briefing. Celebrating milestones and coming together on special days like Christmas and National Days gives people the opportunity to feel the event is more than just a run or walk, but something bigger they are part of. After 20 years, there is usually something to celebrate every week at every event, whether that is a regular having a birthday, a couple joining in on the morning of their wedding day, or a big milestone being reached by a participant or volunteer. These celebrations are encouraged by people bringing cakes or treats to the finish, running in fancy dress or with balloons, or popping open a bottle of Champagne at the finish line. Some parkruns might organise a Guard of Honour to celebrate a special person finishing, and most continue the celebrations online by sharing pictures and details of milestones on event social media pages. Research has shown this kind of social cohesion is key to people keeping up with exercise. A study published in 2018 on the health benefits of parkrun found that 'the supportive environment, positive atmosphere, and sense of belonging are key facilitators of continued

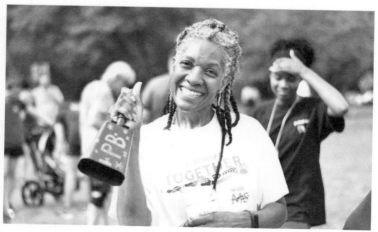

Ringing the Personal Best bell

participation at parkrun, particularly amongst those who have not been previously active'.

Melanie Gearing, a practice manager of a GP surgery, which is part of the parkrun practice initiative, has done 360 parkruns at 110 venues. She loves her parkrun community so much she wanted to include it in her wedding day in 2017. To invite all participants as guests would have proven quite expensive so instead she had a mock wedding at her home parkrun in Huntingdon before the actual ceremony.

Melanie, 51, said : 'I love how my local parkrun brings my friends from many different places together all at the same time. So when my husband-to-be, Cy, and I got engaged, I just knew that my love of parkrun had to be an integral part of our wedding day. We purposefully booked our ceremony on a Saturday at 3pm so that we had plenty of time to do the parkrun first. The table plan at the reception had a parkrun theme. Our big day was advertised on Huntington parkrun's social media pages inviting everyone to come to the parkrun that morning dressed up. Cy and I wore bride and groom outfits and our friends dressed up as guests. The RD that day dressed up as a vicar and added lines from a typical wedding ceremony eg "we are gathered here today..." to the usual briefing which kept everyone entertained. I always find parkrun the best way to start the weekend with friends, and this was the best way to start our wedding day!'

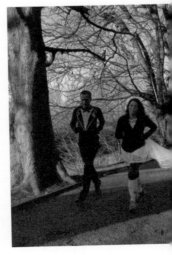

parkrun wedding! Melanie and Cy Gearing

While many like Melanie love how the parkrun community helps them celebrate good times, for others like Louise Liddle, it has offered comfort and solace in very sad

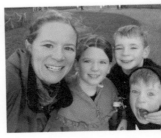

Louise Liddle and her family

DID YOU KNOW?

If it doesn't fall on a Saturday, individual parkruns are allowed to put on an additional event on January 1st each year to celebrate the new year.

times. Her husband, John, died suddenly in 2023 after he was hit by a bus when cycling home from playing football. John, a father to their two boys, James, nine, and Ewan, seven, loved to participate in Chopwell parkrun, Gateshead, so Louise thought it would be wonderful to honour his memory there. On a Saturday in November 2023, the event became a 'Run for John' Staff from where he worked at Virgin Money joined in, helped fill the volunteer roster, and provided a buffet at the finish, while James and Ewan, who had previously only taken part in junior parkruns, completed the 5k for the first time.

Louise, 40, a senior programme manager in education, recalls: 'We were truly grateful for the support we received from the parkrun community that day. Positivity shone through for the first time since we'd not had John in our lives. It felt wonderful to be able to celebrate him with friends and family. A lot of John's running club and other friends turned out too who wanted to support us but didn't know how. There were 134 finishers, one of the biggest turnouts in Chopwell's history. It was a positive experience as we grieved, especially for the boys, who enjoyed running the 5k. Since then, I have regularly taken the boys along to volunteer. Grief is such a strange journey and I find it helps them to connect with nature and people, and to be part of making something happen. They continue to regularly take part in the Riverside junior parkrun in County Durham too.'

BENEFITS FOR CHILDREN

Just as with adults, exercise has numerous benefits for the health, well-being and development of children. Children who are active have improved cardiorespiratory and muscular fitness, better bone and mental health, and have been found to perform better at school. The

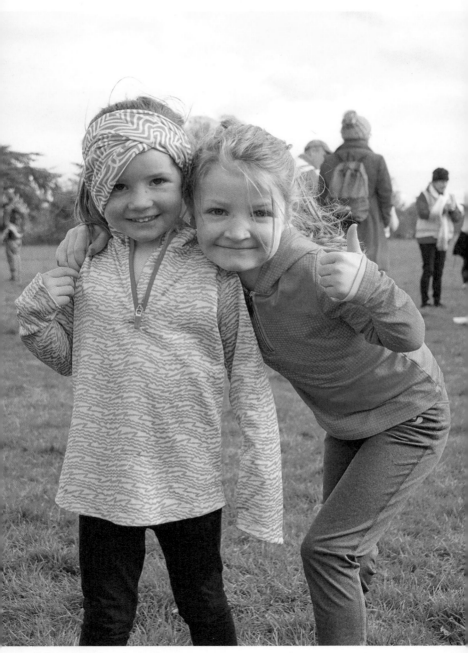

Children give parkrun the thumbs up

WHO recommends children and teens aged 5-17 should do at least 60 minutes per day of moderate-to-vigorous intensity activity across the week. But many globally fall short of this target. junior parkruns (and parkruns for older children and teens) offer an ideal opportunity for them to gain this exercise in a safe, fun environment.

Participating in junior parkruns and parkruns gives them goals to work towards (achieving milestones and faster times) and teaches them resilience if they ever don't run as well as they hoped. It also gets them out in nature, socialising with others and spending time with their family. Getting children involved in exercise they enjoy means they will see it as a pleasure and not a chore, so they will be more likely to continue doing it and reaping the health benefits into adulthood. A 2023 study of junior parkrun in Australia found a near majority of the children who took part (91 per cent) said they found it enjoyable. Of those who responded to the survey, 90 per cent said parkrun 'was fun', while 85 per cent said it was 'energising' and 70 per cent 'challenging' The study concluded that

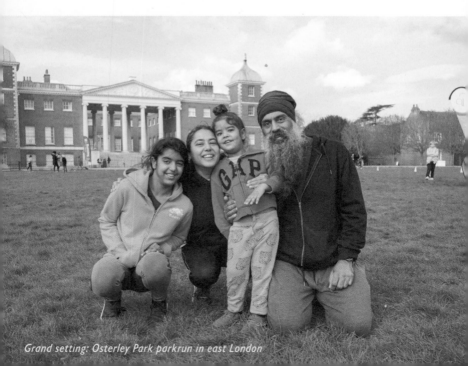

Grand setting: Osterley Park parkrun in east London

junior parkrun has huge promise for 'enabling children to engage in physical activity, in their local communities in a fun and inclusive way' and that it can 'specifically target those not participating in any sports, given the high levels of enjoyment in a non-competitive, non-team environment.'

These children certainly agree. Aggie Gaunt, 10, who has run 58 times at Rushcliffe junior parkrun in Nottingham says: 'I love it because it inspires me to run faster each week and make improvements.' She has improved so much she was the first finisher overall on one occasion. Her brother, Rafe, 9, is also a big fan having participated in 56: 'I enjoy it, especially when it is muddy. It is fun to run first thing in the morning.' Autumn Whitehead, 8, is another keen junior parkrunner at Rushcliffe. She says: 'I love parkrun because I love seeing how many people I can run past and then seeing if I got a PB. I love having a hot chocolate afterwards too, if it is a cold day.'

Meanwhile, Dylan Blake, 5, who is already quite the parkrun tourist having participated in numerous junior events at Rushcliffe, as well as Cassiobury junior parkrun in Watford and Katherine Warington School junior parkrun in Harpenden, says: 'I really like everything about it. I like trying to run faster and I'm excited to get my first wristband once I have done one more. My favourite was on Christmas Eve as I dressed up, there were lots of puddles to jump and Father Christmas gave me a high five!'

Alexa Brooks, 9, who has reached her marathon wristband by doing 22 Riverside junior parkruns in Cambridgeshire, says she 'enjoys seeing if I can improve each week. I just love running!'

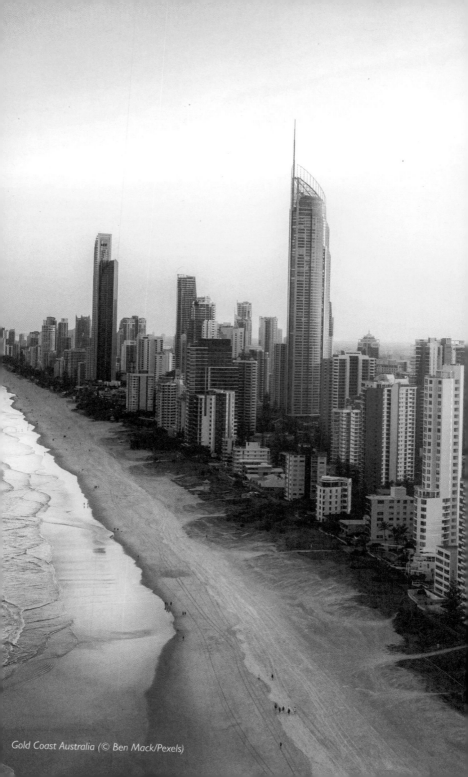

Gold Coast Australia (© Ben Mack/Pexels)

CHAPTER SIX:

PARKRUN AROUND THE WORLD

parkrun continues to gain in growth around the world and can be found in Europe, Asia, Australia, North America and Africa. Many were started by UK expats who wanted to take parkrun with them when they left the country. In other areas it has spread by word of mouth, and people keen to set up an event in their country have contacted parkrun to see if it would be possible.

> **DID YOU KNOW?**
> The first international parkrun was held in Zimbabwe in 2008 but it had to stop running a year later due to political turmoil in the country.

While parkruns around the world all follow the same parkrun code, there are variations in some countries on start times depending on the weather and the daylight. Some are very small in numbers and might have fewer than 20 participants some weeks supported by a small number of volunteers. But all offer the same warm welcome to everyone. Outside of the usual Saturdays, parkrun allows events to be staged on New Year's Day, and one other celebratory day of the country's choice. For some like the UK and Australia, this is Christmas Day, others it is their National Day (eg Canada Day and Malaysia Day) or another day of significance that will usually be a national holiday. These are popular with locals and tourists alike as they are so celebratory with fancy dress and music encouraged.

Here's where you can currently find events outside the UK...

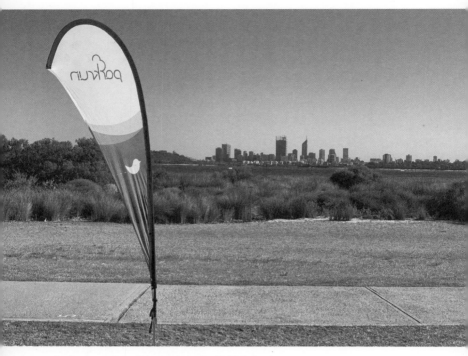

Applecross parkrun, Western Australia (© Chris Barr)

Australia: parkrun has boomed in Australia since the first was held at Main Beach on the Gold Coast back in 2011. Now there are nearly 500 events, including dozens in Tasmania, and a handful of junior parkruns. You're spoilt for choice if you want to run with sea views, as there are numerous around the country's coastline. These include Dolls Point parkrun that runs alongside Botany Bay on the East coast, where Captain Cook famously sailed into Australia in 1770, and Town Beach parkrun in Broome on the West coast, where parkrunners head out and back over the Indian Ocean on Croc Jetty Town Beach Jetty. The coastal parkruns not only offer spectacular views, but a chance to see Australian wildlife, run alongside surfers catching some waves, and have a refreshing post-run dip on a hot morning. You can also run through a vineyard at Ocean View parkrun, or along dusty red paths through native bushland at Cloncurry parkrun, both in Queensland. At Cobram parkrun, Victoria, you might spot a koala as you run along the picturesque route by the Murray River, while kangaroos are often spectators at events including Westerfolds parkrun in Melbourne. For those who like a challenge, Mundy Regional parkrun, Kalamunda, is all on trail and climbs 215 metres. As a result, the average finish time there is 41:33, compared to the national average in Australia of 33:16. There are numerous options which allow you to see the sights in the big cities of Melbourne, Sydney and Perth. Some of these like Albert parkrun in Melbourne attract huge numbers – their record attendance is 1090 with 685 on average. Due to the warm and tropical temperatures, start times deviate from the UK standard of 9am, with many Australian parkruns getting going at 7, 7.30 or 8am. Don't forget to thank the 'vollies' as volunteers are known as Down Under.

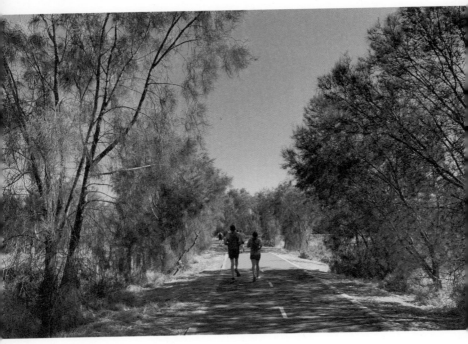

Canning River parkrun, Western Australia (© Chris Barr)

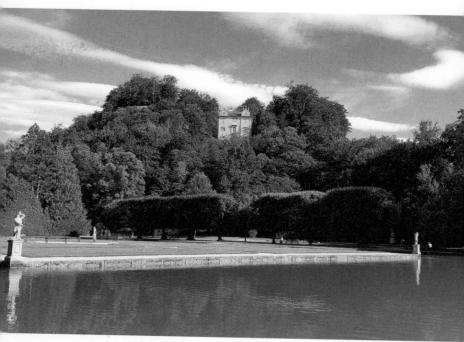

Hellbrunn, Salzburg (© DanyB/Pexels)

Austria: parkrun is relatively new to Austria having only started there in 2021. There are currently only four events spread across the country including Donaupark parkrun in the capital of Vienna, which has PB potential with its flat, lapped route on tarmac with views of the Danube Tower. The Danube cycle path parkrun in Linz, and City Park parkrun, in Graz, are also flat, fast courses, contributing to the average finishing time in the country being 29:17. Hellbrunn parkrun in Salzburg is a must visit for fans of The Sound of Music, as it is the home of the summer house where the song '16 going on 17' was filmed.

Canada: Following the launch in 2016, there are now 47 events. A number of these are in the cities of Toronto, Ottawa and Vancouver, then others are scattered around the country in some stunningly beautiful locations, including Corner Brook Stream Trail parkrun in Newfoundland. Most are on trails and many on some hilly routes, making the average finishing time in Canada 32:43. parkrunners around the country may spot the local wildlife including coyotes, skunks, racoons, and bald eagles – but will hope to avoid encountering any bears. Millennium parkrun in Alberta is a must-visit for parkrun adventurers who can then go on to further explore the famous Banff National park in the Canadian Rockies. Watch out for the 'one hill' RDs joke about on the course of Chain of Lakes parkrun in Nova Scotia – you run down and then back up it on the out and back route. The country's furthest North is Birchwood Trails parkrun near Fort McMurray, a popular area for hiking through a boreal forest. Over on the West coast, Clover Point parkrun on Vancouver Island is on an oceanfront course with magnificent views over the water.

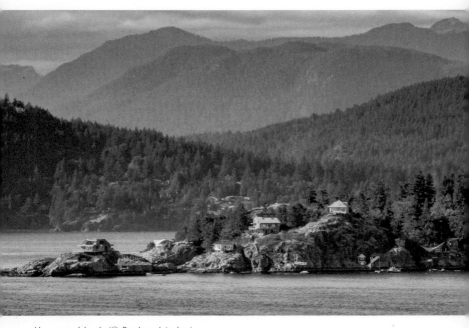

Vancouver Islands (© Pat Josse/pixabay)

Denmark: Amager Fælled parkrun was launched in Copenhagen in 2009, making it the longest-standing parkrun (and Denmark the longest-standing parkrun territory) outside the UK. However, since then parkrun's growth in the Scandinavian country has been small. There are still only nine events and four of them are in the capital. Amager Strandpark is one of Copenhagen's most popular with its sea views across The Sound to Sweden (where Malmö Ribersborg parkrun takes place on the other side of the Øresund Bridge). Numbers soar on the public holiday of Ascension Day when tourists often join in for the fancy dress and party atmosphere. Elsewhere in the country, the events are low key with a small number of participants and a handful of volunteers. Some use flour to mark out the course in the absence of marshals, as it doesn't need to be cleared away afterwards: it will be eaten by the birds or washed away in the rain. The furthest North is Nibe parkrun, an area famed for its annual music festival and 'Hollywood letters' spelling out Nibe. parkrunners pass the letters as well as passing through a forest on the slightly hilly route. The majority of the parkruns in the country are flat and fast, giving a speedy average finishing time of 26:35 – the fastest average of all global parkruns.

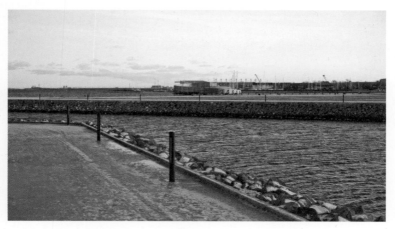

Amager Strandpark: site of the longest-running parkrun outside the UK (© Monica Hassel/Flikr)

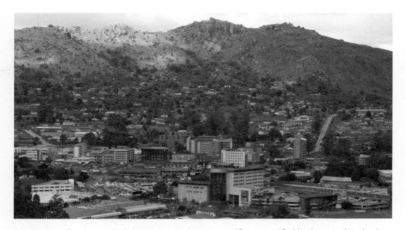

Mbabane in Eswatini, which hosts two parkruns on golf courses (© Mimkreative/pixabay)

Eswatini: There are just two events in this landlocked African country. The first, Mbabane parkrun, has been running since 2017 around the picturesque Mbabane golf course in Eswatini and attracts 68 attendees on average. It has a speedy course record of 14.56 but the average finishing time is 37.29. Manzini parkrun followed in 2022, also around a golf course, but smaller in numbers with just 16 a week on average, and a slower average finishing time of 40:02. Volunteering here is popular, with some weeks the number of volunteers exceeding or equalling the number of participants. Both have 8am starts to beat the heat (and presumably the golfers to the course).

Finland: Since launching in the country in 2017 with Tampere parkrun, there are now a total of seven events, starting at the later time of 9.30am. Most take place on picturesque routes alongside water, including Tokoinranta parkrun around Toolo Bay in Helsinki, an out and back route providing lovely views of the City. Lahti port parkrun is another with beautiful watery views beside Vesijärvi Lake along a beach boulevard. Running on compacted snow is common at some locations in the winter months so the average finishing time is 33:36. Finland's claim to parkrun fame is

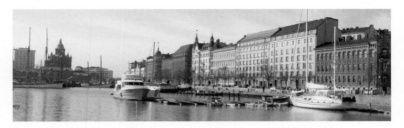

Helsinki waterfront: parkrunners are greeted with stunning views (© reijotelaranta/pixabay)

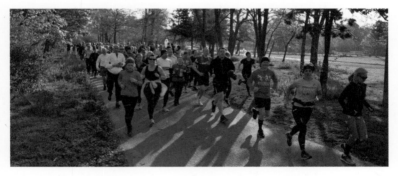

parkrun in Paris, before the event was suspended (© Laurent Dessirier/Flikr)

that it is home to the most northerly event in the world. Pokkinen parkrun in Oulu is just below the Arctic Circle – read more about it in the global bucket list.

France: Between 2017 and 2022, there were eight popular parkruns in France, in places including Paris, Bordeaux and Rouen. However, they never returned after parkrun was suspended globally following the Covid19 pandemic. In France, it is now mandatory for those participating in sporting activities to have an official medical certif-icate from a doctor. This made it impossible for parkrun to continue as it doesn't have the resources to enforce this rule, and it goes against its ethos of making exercise accessible to everyone as it creates a barrier to participation. parkrun is trying to work with the French authorities to find a solution, so events may return in France one day.

Germany: parkrun launched here in 2017 with three simultaneous runs in Hannover, Leipzig and Mannheim. These events were the first to test the parkrun Virtual Volunteer app, which has allowed parkruns across the world to operate more efficiently with less equipment. Germans quickly embraced parkrun and more and more started across the country, offering the chance to run on various routes including through woodlands, around lakes and reservoirs and within big cities including Frankfurt and Osnabruck. There are now 59 events and counting, with an average finishing time of 30:30 . Hasenheide parkrun is popular with visitors to the capital of Berlin, and numbers soar when it is marathon weekend as many opt to take part for a pre-26.2 mile 'shake out' run. Meanwhile many tourists like to time a visit to West Park parkrun in Munich with their famous Oktoberfest. Ziegelwiese parkrun in Halle offers a way for alphabet hunters to get a coveted 'Z', but few seem to make the trip as the average attendance each week is only 16. parkrunners at Rosenstein Park parkrun in Stuttgart might spot some wild animals as the route passes the city's zoo, while at Riemer parkrun in Munich you could 'land' yourself a PB, as it is on a former airport runway.

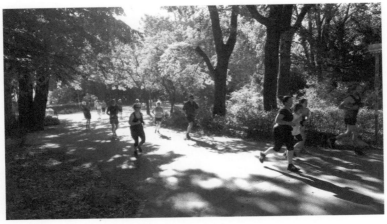

Hasenheide parkrun in Berlin: popular with tourists (© Aljoscha Marcel Everding/Flikr)

Ireland: parkrun has been thriving in the Republic of Ireland since 2012 and there are currently 110 events, plus 35 junior parkruns spread across the country. Events here start at the later time of 9.30am. There are a number around Dublin including Father Collins parkrun, where you pass wetlands flanked by wind turbines and a striking waterfall feature. Malahide parkrun, near Dublin, was the country's very first event and continues to attract nearly 300 people each week who love the route in the grounds of a castle dating back to the 12th century. Many of Ireland's coastal parkruns offer spectacular views of the Irish Sea and the Atlantic Ocean. Bere Island parkrun, off the coast of Cork, is one of the most breathtaking with additional views of a Viking harbour and requires a ferry crossing to get there from the mainland (as does Inis Meáin parkrun — see the global bucket list for more on this one). If you want an extra challenge, tackle the sand dunes at Erris parkrun in County Mayo, which has an average finishing time of 34:30, more than four minutes slower than the national average of 30:16. Meanwhile, Rostrevor parkrun in Kilbroney Park, Rostrevor, has a bit of everything on the route taking participants along a riverside trail, through a forest and a hay meadow with views of Carlingford Lough. The area was often visited by C.S. Lewis and inspired his books, so you also pass through a 'door to Narnia.'

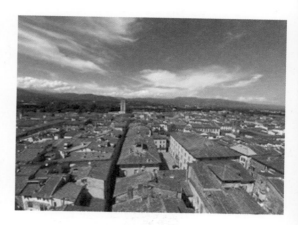

Beautiful view from the Lucca parkrun in Italy.
(© Adrian Pattison)

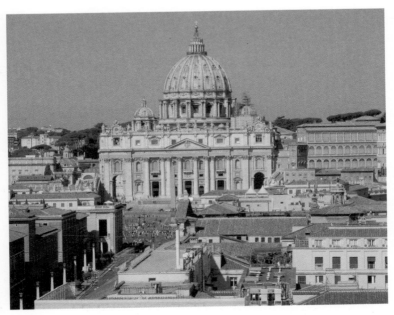

St Peter's Basilica in Rome: parkrun arrived in Italy in 2015 (© ptra/pixabay)

Italy: The first Italian parkrun to launch was Uditore parkrun in Palermo, Sicily, back in 2015, which had just five finishers and nine volunteers. While numbers continue to be on the low side each week, with 32 attendees on average, there is a big appetite for parkrun in the area and two more followed in Palermo – Favorita parkrun and Foro Italico – making it a good spot for anyone who wants to tick off a couple of parkrun locations while on a holiday. parkrunners have the rare opportunity to run on an active volcano, as Etna parkrun is held at the foot of the mountain. There are 14 events in total in Italy, with an average finishing time of 30:59. Outside of Sicily, these can mostly be found near the big cities including Milan and Venice. Caffarella parkrun and Roma Pineto parkrun are both in Rome, with the latter offering beautiful views of St. Peter's basilica. Meanwhile, the Walls of Lucca parkrun is a must-visit for many. See the bucket list of global parkruns to find out why.

Japan: Running is popular in Japan and there are now 37 parkruns spread across the islands with an average finishing time of 32:32. Here you can parkrun with stunning mountain and sea views, and under the country's famous blossom trees in the Spring. It started in 2019 with Futakotamagawa parkrun, Tokyo, and there are now a number of others around the capital. These include Urayasu City General Park parkrun that is on a palm-tree lined seafront route close to Disneyland, while the off-road Ome Hills parkrun follows an undulating hiking trail and has views of Mount Fuji on a clear day. Central park parkrun is Japan's furthest North in Morioka City, where parkrunners have spectacular views of Mount Iwate. For some Japanese history, visit Heijo Palace Ruins Historical Park parkrun in Nara, which was the ancient capital of Japan. The parkrun loops this significant UNESCO World Heritage site, where sights include a reconstruction of the striking Former Audience Hall which was once used for important ceremonies. Meanwhile, there are four parkruns to choose from on the lush island of Shikoku, including Horinouchi koen parkrun in Matsuyama City, at the foot of Matsuyama Castle built in 1603.

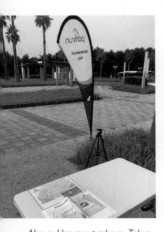

Above: Urayasu parkrun, Tokyo, Japan (© Nick Buttenshaw)

Below: Cherry blossoms in Morioka City (© Tagosaku/Flikr)

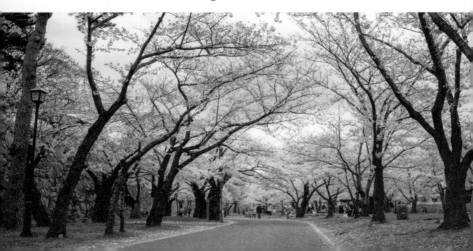

Malaysia: Presint 18 parkrun, in Putrajaya, launched in Malaysia in 2018. The out and back route along Putrajaya Lake starts at 7.30am and is regularly well-attended with an average of 87 runners, with an average finishing time of 41:05. This is currently the only parkrun in Malaysia as the popular Taman Pudu Ulu parkrun in Cheras had to cease running in 2022 after four years, as an agreement could not be reached with the landowner for it to continue.

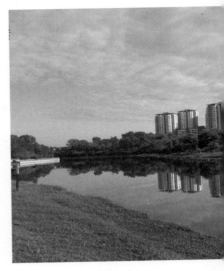

Presint 18 parkrun in Malaysia (© Soong-Kong Au Yeong)

Namibia: There are currently three scenic events in Namibia. The first — Swakopmund parkrun — was launched in April 2017 in a beautiful seafront location that continues to attract 78 parkrunners on average each week. Walvis Bay parkrun followed slightly further down the coast in 2018. Here a flamboyance of flamingos are regular spectators, as the route runs alongside a flamingo lagoon. Further inland, Windhoek parkrun, held on a golf course where you might spot a mongoose, completed the country's parkrun trio in 2019. Many choose to walk rather than run, making the average finishing time across the country 41:50.

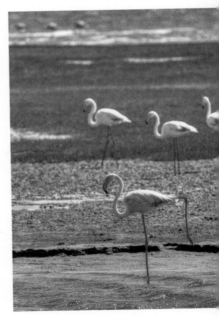

Flamingos at Walvis Bay, Namibia (© Nicolas Rénac/Flikr)

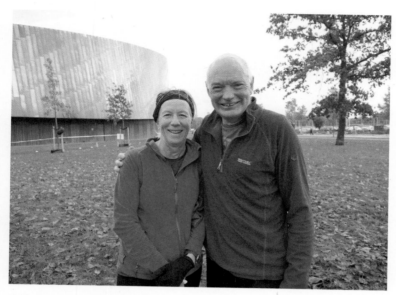

Zuiderpark parkrun, Netherlands – popular with Z-hunters!

Netherlands: Such was the appetite for parkrun in the Netherlands, six launched on the same day in 2020. It's quickly grown and there are now 23 events across the country with more in the offing. In Amsterdam, Amsterdamse Bos parkrun can be found in the southern outskirts of the city. It's a flat, one lap route around a large tranquil forest and attracts 161 participants on average. Many cycle to get there. Kagerzoom parkrun in Warmond is one which offers views of the country's famous windmills, as does Kralingse Bos parkrun in Rotterdam. This takes participants on a scenic route through a forest and then alongside a lake. Zuiderpark parkrun in The Hague and Zegerplas parkrun in Alphen aan den Rijn provide alphabet hunters with two beautiful ways to gain their Z on their picturesque routes. With mostly flat routes, the nation's average finishing time is quicker than many others around the world, at 29:40.

New Zealand: parkrun was launched in New Zealand with Lower Hutt parkrun in Wellington in 2012. There are now 46 events across the North and South islands and it is hoped that in the near future, they could reach 100 locations. There are plenty of pretty options to choose from in the cities of Auckland and Wellington, and no shortage of stunning routes further afield in the country. To name a few: Queenstown parkrun in Queenstown offers a pine forest, lake path and views of snow-capped mountains; at Wanaka parkrun in Wanaka you can glimpse the area's famous Wanaka Tree as you run around the sparkling lake; and at Puarenga Park parkrun in Rotorua who can run on a sulphur track in the region's rare geothermal field. Many of the country's events stagger their start times based on the season – so they are held at 8am in the summer and 9am in the winter. The average finishing time is 31:51.

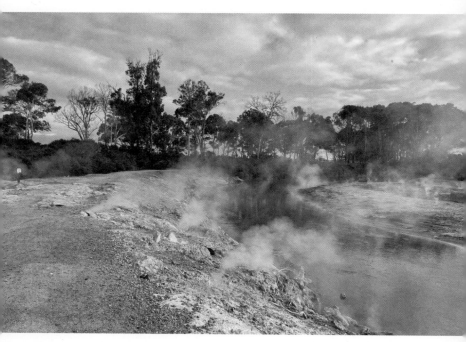

The sulphur track at Puarenga Park parkrun, New Zealand (© Richard Derrick)

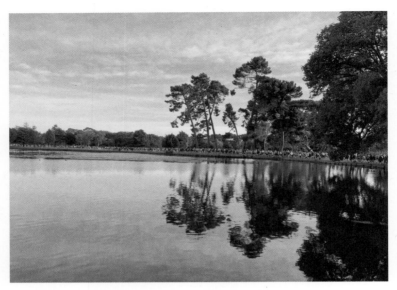

Hagley parkrun, Christchurch, New Zealand (© Richard Derrick)

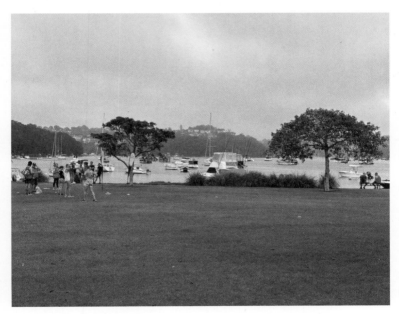

Mosman parkrun in New Zealand: also offers good views (© Johanna Houlahan)

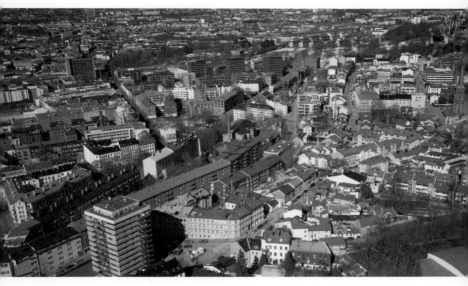

View of Oslo from Tøyen (Wikimedia Commons)

Norway: There are currently just seven events around the country – and most of them are best described as hilly. Burning quads are rewarded with panoramic scenes of the stunning Norwegian landscape. Tøyen parkrun – the country's first parkrun launched in August 2017 – has amazing views of Oslo (another in the capital city – Ekebergsletta parkrun – followed in 2022) while Løvstien parkrun climbs a gravel path up Mount Løvstakken for views of the city of Bergen, its surrounding mountains and the North Sea. Further north, Festningen parkrun is held on elevated trails around a fortress. Meanwhile, Stavanger parkrun in Rogaland offers sweeping views of Stavanger and lake Mosvatnet, but you have to brave a steep hill which has been coined 'Mount Doom' first. Sterkfontein parkrun, Skien, also involves a tough incline up into a forest, which on average only nine participants climb each week. Locals are used to hiking the technical ups and downs of the mountains so despite the elevation on many courses, the average finishing time is 29:00.

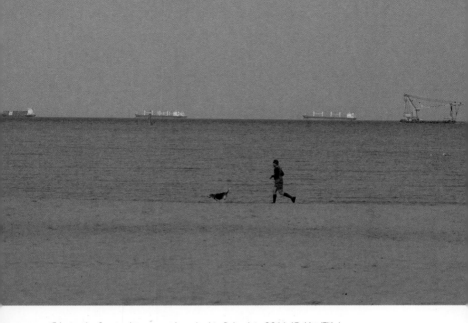

Gdynia: the first parkrun event launched in Poland, in 2011 (© Usz/Flikr)

Poland: This is another thriving parkrun territory with 95 events, and an average finishing time of 28:35. The first was Gdynia parkrun launched in 2011 on the country's north coast, which had just five participants back then. Now it has grown to 87 on average each week enjoying the route along a promenade by the Baltic Sea. Other locations are spread across the country with a handful in big cities including Warsaw and Krakow. At Cieszyn parkrun in the South West, you actually pass into the Czech Republic when running on one side of the Olza River. In November, parkruns celebrate Poland's Independence Day creating a sea of red and white as participants are encouraged to wear their national colours and carry flags. Those looking to complete their Alphabets are well catered for in Poland, as there are a number to choose from starting with the letter Z: Zielony Jar parkrun just outside Krakow; Zalew Żyrardowski parkrun in central Poland; Zamek w Malborku parkrun in Malbork (see more on this in the global bucket run list), and Zielona Góra parkrun, a forest route in the city of the same name in Western Poland.

Singapore: There are three events here popular with locals and tourists who often squeeze in a parkrun while stopping over en route flying to other destinations. All start at 7.30am in hot and humid conditions being so close to the equator. The first was East Coast parkrun, which has grown from 36 people at the first event to an average of 127 today. Participants can enjoy an out and back route along the picturesque coastline as the sun rises over the Singapore Strait. Over on the west coast, West Coast Park parkrun is a figure of eight loop in a waterfront park where parrots fly overhead and children love the giant playground. The third, Bishan parkrun, is inland and runs parallel to the Kallang River in Bishan-Ang Mo Kio Park on tarmac footpaths. You might spot wildlife like otters and herons. While the climate can be challenging, none of the courses are so the average finishing time across them is 29:10.

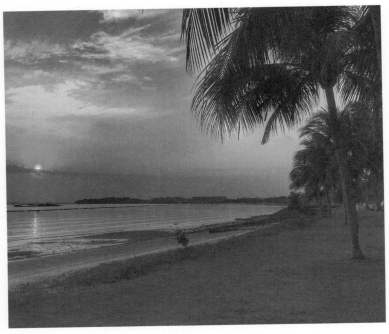

Sunrise: all parkruns in Singapore start at 7.30am(© cattan2011/Flikr)

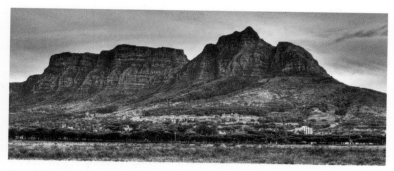

View of Table Mountain from Rondebosch common (© Hubert January/Flikr)

South Africa: As founder Paul Sinton-Hewitt is from South Africa, he was keen to take it to his homeland. Time Trials are already popular in the country so parkrun was an easy sell and an instant hit. The first event was Delta parkrun in Johannesburg in 2011. There are now 219 to choose from, varying from coastal locations to those in the desert and in the foothills of mountains. You don't need to go on a safari when you're a parkrunner in the country, as you might encounter giraffes at Hluluwe parkrun, or spot a pride of lions at Nkomazi parkrun, near Tonga village, to the south of Kruger National Park. There are a number in and around Cape Town, including Zandvlei parkrun for those completing an Alphabet Challenge. Rondebosch Common parkrun has a backdrop of Table Mountain and Devil's Peak, while you also get great views of the famous mountains from Melkbosstrand and Big Bay parkruns (for more on the latter see the global bucket list). In Johannesburg, there's a plethora of parkruns: Wits parkrun is around a university; Zuurfontein parkrun is a busy 'Z' option with 207 participants each week on average; and Meyers Farm parkrun is a scenic trail route past stables of horses. Elsewhere, South Africa is also home to the delightfully named Piggly Wiggly parkrun, in Howick, an undulating route which zig zags through a vineyard, and Dullstroom parkrun in the Dullstroom Nature Reserve, Mpumalanga, which has one of the highest elevations of parkruns around the world at 2,100m. Roses parkrun outside Pretoria goes around a nursery of roses, which offer a beautiful background when in flower. Almost 30 percent of those completing a parkrun each week in South Africa are walkers, the highest figure of all the parkrun countries, making the average finishing time 41:50.

Sweden: Another Scandinavian country in the parkrun family with 11 events. Three of these are near Stockholm, including Haga parkrun which was the first to launch in the capital in 2016. The pretty course is two laps around a forest and lake with striking architecture to be seen including the Chinese Temple, the Turkish Kiosk, and Haga Palace. Another near Stockholm is Huddinge parkrun, held in a forest popular with hikers which is described as 'very hilly'. Skatås parkrun in Gothenburg is another hilly one but anyone struggling with the inclines can distract themselves by taking in views of the serene Härlanda Tjärn the course loops around. Most of Sweden's parkruns safely go ahead on compacted snow during the winter, which doesn't slow down most participants as the average finishing time in the country is

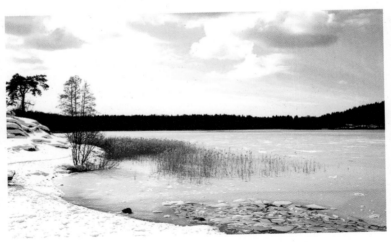

Härlanda Tjärn: an atmsopheric parkrun in Sweden (Wikimedia Commons)

swift at 28:41. However, Broparken parkrun in Umeå – the second most northerly parkrun in the world behind Finland's Pokkinen parkrun – doesn't run from early December to April because the sub zero temperatures make it too dangerous for the volunteers, and only 14 attend on average during warmer periods.

USA: It is fair to say parkrun has not had a huge surge in growth in the USA despite being present in the vast country for more than a decade. The first event launched in the country was Livonia parkrun, Michigan, in 2012, which was also the first parkrun in the Western Hemisphere. Word soon spread in

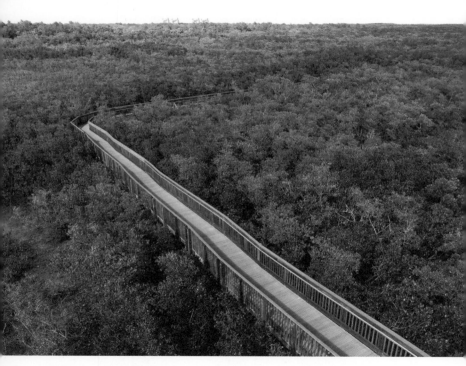

parkrunners at the Weedon Island Preserve parkrun, Florida, run along these boardwalks surrounded by mangroves (© Michael Barbosa)

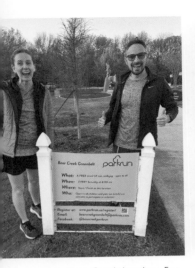
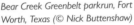

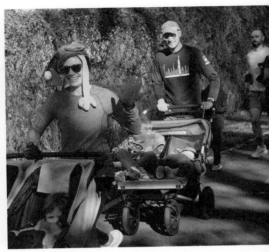

Bear Creek Greenbelt parkrun, Fort Worth, Texas (© Nick Buttenshaw)

Thanksgiving parkrun, College Park, Maryland (© phillips_colin/Flikr)

this area and there are now three additional parkruns within 16 miles of one another. Across the country, there are now 66 events in total, spread far and wide across the East to West coast in mountains, around lakes, through forests, and in tranquil green spaces in densely populated urban areas. Many states are yet to have a parkrun, and some like California have just one – that's Byxbee parkrun north of San Jose centre. In the cities of Seattle, Washington DC, Detroit and Boston you can find multiple options but some of the country's most visited cities including New York, Los Angeles and Miami remain parkrun-less. The USA can lay claim to having the highest parkrun in the world. Aspen parkrun in Colorado is held at 2,400m above sea level. The average finishing time there is 32:20, which is actually quicker than the country's national average of 33:58, despite the altitude. Start times vary from state to state but all aim to celebrate Thanksgiving with a special event where participants are encouraged to dress up as turkeys!

TEN OF THE BEST GLOBAL PARKRUNS FOR TOURISTS' BUCKET LISTS

parkruns in all parts of the world feature breathtaking views, standout features and the chance to be immersed in beautifully untouched landscapes. So it is difficult to choose just 10 locations. Consider this selection of particularly interesting venues a starting point for your wanderlust…

1. Hamilton Island parkrun, Australia: This idyllic island in the Whitsundays is a dream destination for many. It is famed for its crystal blue seas, soft, white sandy beaches and the Great Barrier Reef below its surrounding waters. parkrun started here in 2015 but as it

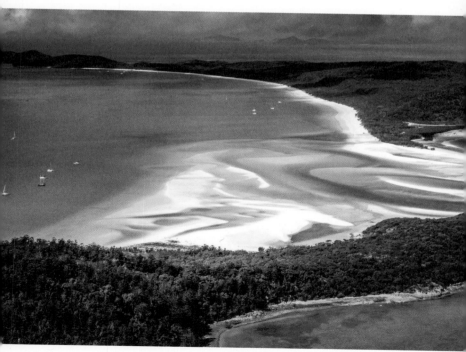

Hamilton Island offers a parkrun in paradise (© Russell Charters/Flikr)

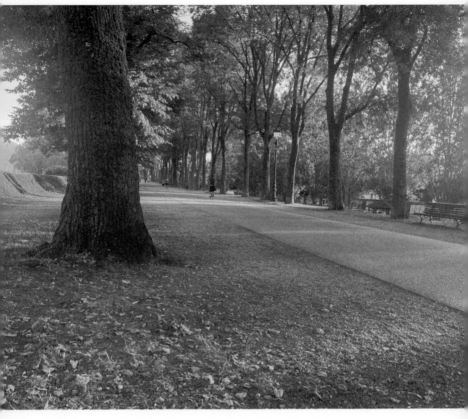

The path on the walls, Walls of Lucca parkrun, Italy (© Jenny Maginley)

is a private island, attendance is often low at 33 participants, with four volunteers on average. Those joining in are treated to a route with unbeatable views as they run past 'Shady Creek' lawn and the 'Scenic Trail' entrance onto the palm-tree lined Catseye Beach, overlooking the sparkling turquoise waters of Catseye Bay. The run starts at 7am as the sun rises over the lush green surrounding hills. Finishing times vary depending on whether there is a high or low tide on the 2k beach section. The average finish time is 31.30 so don't visit for a PB but to soak up the location of this parkrun in paradise.

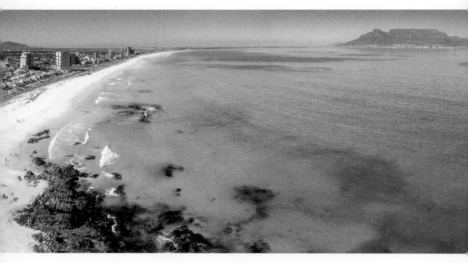

The jaw-dropping scenery at Big Bay, Cape Town, in South Africa (Wikimedia Commons)

2. Mura di Lucca parkrun AKA Walls of Lucca parkrun, Italy:
Running on walls surrounding the ancient city is this parkrun's
quirky feature. These walls are the second largest intact example of
a fully walled Renaissance city in Europe (the current ones replace
Medieval and Roman versions). While the walls date back centu-
ries, parkrun has been here since 2018 and is one big loop meaning
parkrunners get to glimpse most of Lucca's sights on their way round,
as well the vibrant green Tuscan hills beyond. The average finishing
time is 31:55 with an average of 61 runners and eight volunteers.

3. Big Bay parkrun, South Africa: Another parkrun with jaw-dropping scenery, the local area is called Eden on the Bay. On the out
and back route along a sandy beach, parkrunners see Robben
Island and enjoy spectacular views of Table Mountain. Breaching
whales and leaping seals are common sights off the coast. The
parkrun here started in 2013 with 46 participants but now attracts
328 a week. The average finishing time is 41:16, due to the soft

sand, and perhaps because people are taking their time to finish to soak up the amazing views.

4. Lake2Lake Trail parkrun, New Zealand: New Zealand abounds with picturesque parkruns, but Lake2Lake in Te Anau on the South Island is special not just for its spectacular lake views, but because it is one of the few parkruns in the world with a number in its title. There's been a parkrun here since 2022 but people have walked and run the trails here for many years, as it is the home of the Kepler track – one of the country's most famous and

Lake2Lake parkrun New Zealand (Carly Webber)

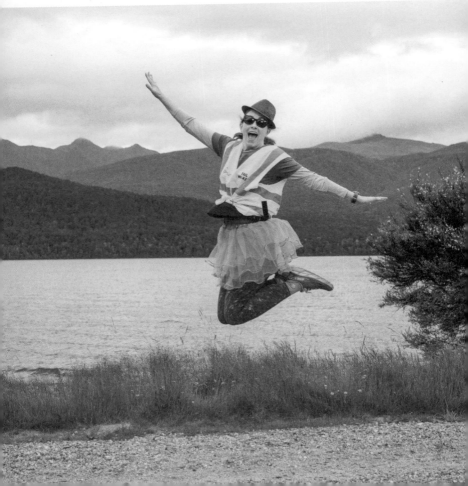

scenic hiking routes that climbs into the mountains of the stunning Fiordland National Park. Some take on running the whole route as part of the Kepler Challenge ultra race. parkrunners experience a Fiordland 'gentle rise' (AKA hill) as they go along the route's gravel path before turning back into the Te Anau bird park. Here, they might spot the endangered flightless bird, Takahe. The undulating route means the average finishing time is 36.35 for a turnout of 32 participants and eight volunteers (on average).

5. Inis Meáin parkrun, Ireland: Another parkrun on a small island but this one couldn't be more different to the Australian option on this list. Inis Meáin parkrun is held on the island of the same name which is one of the Aran Islands off Ireland's west coast. It has a beautiful rugged landscape and vast views across the Atlantic ocean. parkrun only started on the island – which has a population of about 200 people – in 2023. The average attendance is only 27 with an average of eight volunteers. Non-resident participants have

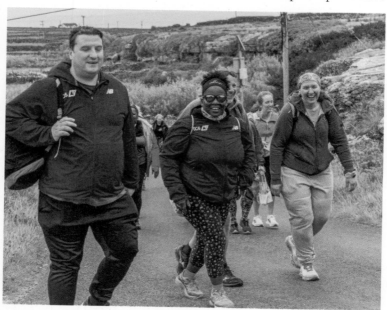

Walking parkrun at Inis Meáin, amid the rugged landscape of Ireland's West Coast

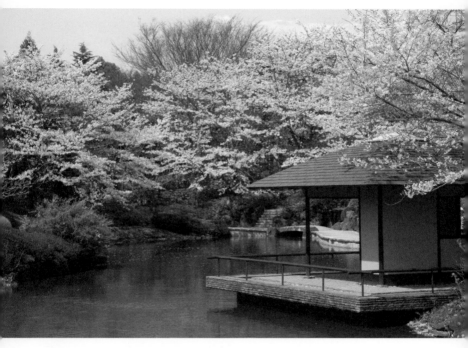

Kashiwanoha park in Chiba: a tranquil green space in Tokyo (© autan/Flikr)

time to catch a ferry from the mainland in the morning, as this run begins at 11am. This is to allow islanders to attend morning mass, as they have to share their priest with the two other Aran islands. The undulating two lap route is entirely on public roads lined with stone walls. Thankfully, there is hardly any traffic. But the uphill sections slow the average finishing time to 37:53. Participants have plenty of scenic sea views as they walk/run and can enjoy some Irish hospitality afterwards in the community hall for a post-run coffee.

6. *Kashiwanoha parkrun, Japan:* Many parkruns offer an oasis of nature within a more built up area and this is the case with Kashiwanoha park in Chiba. The tranquil green space, surrounded by buildings including those of Tokyo University, includes a serene duck pond and a beautiful rose garden. You can track the seasons via its

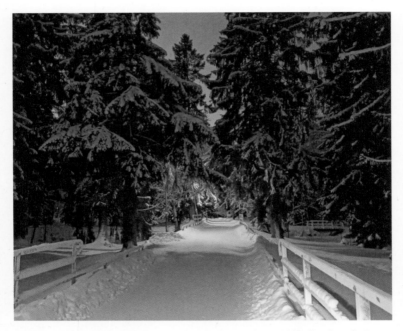

Pokkinen parkrun in Finland: the most northerly parkrun in the world (© Chris Beresford)

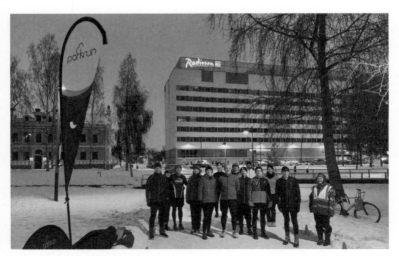

Making the most of the light at Pokkinen park, where the event takes place (© Ville Juutilainen)

abundant trees from the gold and red colours of the oaks and acers in autumn, to the pale pink and white cherry blossoms which are in full bloom in the spring. There's also a tea house within the park where you can experience a traditional Japanese tea ceremony. The parkrun route is three flat loops on concrete paths so has plenty of PB potential, making the average finishing time 28:17. It has been running here since 2019 with numbers steadily rising so the number of participants is 61, with 11 volunteers on average.

7. Pokkinen parkrun, Finland: If you want to run in a winter wonderland, then Pokkinen parkrun in Oulu (the capital of northern Scandinavia) is the place. It is the most northerly parkrun in the world – with freezing temperatures and little daylight in the winter. It starts at 9.30am which is before sunrise from late November to January. In the summer, the route, alongside the Oulujoki River and the Gulf of Bothnia, offers beautiful views of

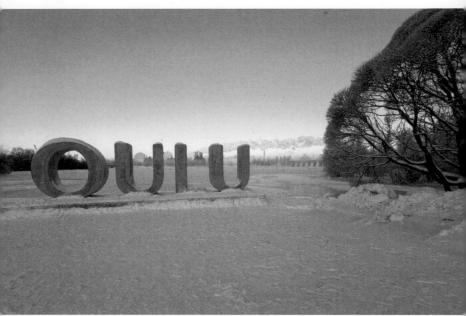

Pokkinen parkrun takes place in Oulu, a city in Finland (© Sampo Valjus)

the water glimmering in the sun. The course is flat but the average time of 30:19 is slowed by the snow in the cold months. There are also a lot of bridges to cross – 14 in total – including one over a dam. About 20 people a week have attended this run close to the Arctic Circle since it started in 2021, helped by an average of five hardy volunteers. Numbers rise in the Spring and Summer, along with the sun.

8. Cape Pembroke Lighthouse parkrun, Falklands: At the other end of the world is Cape Pembroke Lighthouse, near Stanley in the Falkland Islands. It is the world's most southerly parkrun open to the public. There is another slightly further south in the Falklands – Mount Pleasant parkrun – but this takes place on a military base so is only open to authorised people. The Cape Pembroke Light-

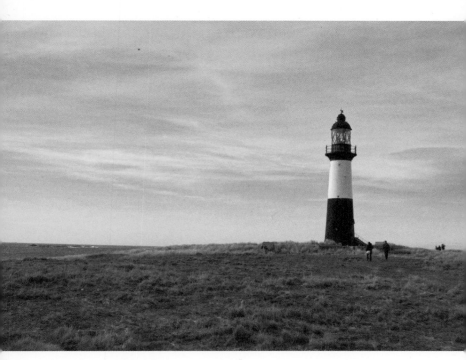

Cape Pembroke Lighthouse: site of the most southerly parkrun in the world open to the public (© Povl Abrahamsen/Flikr)

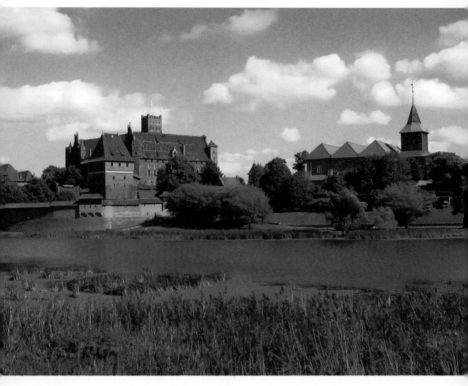

Malbork Castle in Poland: a UNESCO World Heritage site (© Matteo X/Flikr)

house route runs out and back on a gravel path in rocky terrain towards the lighthouse that gives it its name. It was launched in 2019 and has an average finish time of 36:47. As the route is on a coastal path, it can be exposed to the elements with no shade on a sunny day and gusty winds at other times but offers amazing views of the surrounding seas where you might spot whales or penguins leaping out of the water. Participation is often on the small side with 19 on average and four volunteers.

9. *Malbork Castle, Poland:* parkrunners run alongside the largest castle in the world (measured by land area) at this UNESCO World Heritage site. Prepare yourself for views of the 13th century fortress, built by the Teutonic Order of knights, on one side and the scenic Nogat River on the other. The course itself is partly run on cobblestones with an average finishing time of 30.11. If the beauty and history of the venue isn't enough to entice you, you'll be pleased to know it will help you complete an alphabet challenge if that is your goal – as its Polish name is Zamek w Malborku parkrun. The flat route was launched in 2019 and has 40 participants and nine volunteers on average. Due to its location in the North of Poland, it can get very snowy in winter. Brrr!

10. Canyon Rim Trail parkrun, USA: This parkrun in Twin Falls, Idaho, is held on the fully paved and scenic Canyon Rim Trail

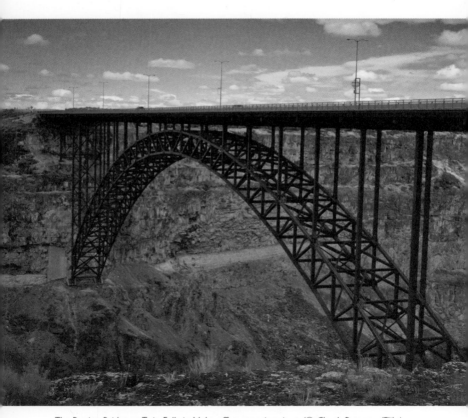

The Perrine Bridge at Twin Falls in Idaho offers stunning views (© Chuck Peterson./Flikr)

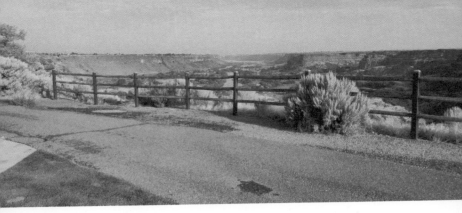

Canyon Rim Trail parkrun route: great for spotting birds of prey (Gerardo Muñoz)

with stunning views of the canyon, waterfalls and Snake River. It is a popular spot for the adventurous, as well as those who enjoy trail walking and cycling. Base jumpers often leap from the Perrine Bridge, which is by the parkrun start, while kayakers love to explore Snake River which the route runs alongside. As it attracts so many outdoorsy people, parkrun started here in 2021 but participation remains low with an average of just 16 participants and five volunteers. The average time is a leisurely 43:11 perhaps because people are spotting birds of prey soaring overhead.

'WHY WE LOVE BEING GLOBAL PARKRUN TOURISTS'

While the majority of parkrunners tend to visit their local (known as 'home' parkrun) the most, and ideally get there by foot, public transport or bike, the growth of so many destinations has led to a boom in so-called 'parkrun tourism'. Many people will travel across the country and the globe specifically to visit a parkrun. Popular destinations are those starting with obscure letters of the alphabet, such as Z, for those trying to complete an A-Z challenge (more on these challenges in Chapter Five), and those held in some of the world's most spectacular locations like in the global bucket list. This tourism can have a benefit on a local economy. Attracting more parkrunners to an area they might not otherwise have visited can lead to them spending money at local businesses and attractions –

and telling their parkrun friends to visit there too. parkrun tourism can help prop up some events too where participation from runners, walkers and volunteers would be significantly lower if only attended by locals.

Anne Kelly, 48, a Data Quality Analyst from Manchester, loves being a parkrun Tourist both in the UK and abroad. She's attended more than 251 parkruns at 124 locations as well as volunteering often. 'I love to travel and parkrun tourism is a great catalyst for visiting new places,' she says. 'parkrun tourism has greatly improved my UK geography and taken me to places I otherwise wouldn't have visited. I find it a great way to motivate myself and gain a sense of achievement. It's also sociable, I love having parkrun day trips/ weekends away with friends and family.'

On one of these trips, Anne managed to do three parkruns within a few days. She first took part in Faelledparken parkrun in Copenhagen on the traditional Saturday, then got to do Amager Strandpark in the city on the Monday, as it was Denmark's Constitution Day when they allow additional parkruns to be held. 'Amager was my favourite overseas event so far. The course around a lagoon was absolutely stunning and there was a real party atmosphere.' Anne and her friends kept the party going by then travelling to Sweden, to attend the Vaxjosjon parkrun, in Vaxjo on Sweden's National Day.

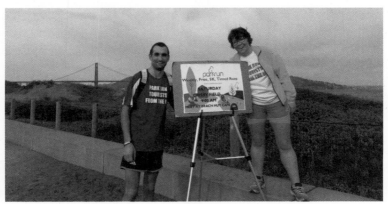

parkrun tourists Pete and Emma Bell in San Francisco

Pete Bell, 42, and his wife, Emma, 46, have done more than 130 parkruns between them in the UK and were keen to experience it in other countries when they went travelling in 2015. They even made 'parkrun tourists from the UK' T-shirts to share their pride in their participation. At Crissy Field parkrun in San Francisco, USA, the pair discovered that parkrun was on a far smaller scale to the UK events they were used to.

Pete, a refit manager from Bury St.Edmunds, recalls: 'We went in our T-shirts expecting to see a bit of excitement that we were visiting from the UK – but the whole event only involved 29 people – and most of them were British tourists or

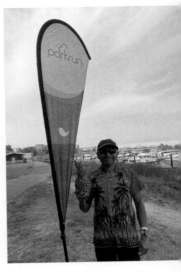

parkrun tourist Arry Nathan running with a pineapple in Canada

expats.' Pete was perplexed about the low numbers as there were many other runners out for solo runs on the same promenade that day, with the backdrop of Alcatraz and the Golden Gate Bridge. The RD told him it was intentionally low key over fears the local council would shut them down if they became too big. Indeed, it did cease running in 2020. Another notable parkrun on the couple's travels was Cairns parkrun, Queensland, Australia. 'The route went out and back along an esplanade and there were warning signs to watch out for crocodiles,' Pete recalls. 'The weather was an experience as well. Half way round we got drenched in a brief tropical downpour, then the sun came back out and we were dry again by the finish line.' Pete said they loved feeling part of the 'parkrun global family' while they were away from home. This is the reason why Arry Nathan, from Nottingham, likes to try and fit in a parkrun while on holiday with his own family. He has been to more than 80 different locations. 'parkrun changed my life,' he admits. 'I wasn't a runner before a friend encouraged me to try one in 2012. Now there's rarely a

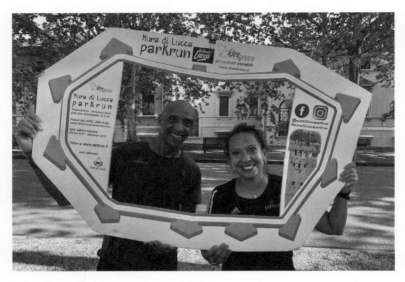

parkrun tourists Errol and Jenny Maginley in Italy

Saturday when I'm not joining in. I don't know how parkrun does it but when I have gone to parkruns in other countries, they've had the same homely feel as the ones I've done in the UK. The vibe of friendliness and inclusivity is always there.' Arry took a unique element of his home parkrun in Colwick, Nottingham, with him to Canada in 2023. Colwick parkrun hold an 'Hawaiian shirt' themed day every summer where everyone dresses up and there are records for those who run the fastest carrying a piece of fruit. 'My friend Steve Shanks loved parkrun and held the record for carrying a pineapple. He died in 2023 after taking part in the London Marathon so at Richmond Olympic parkrun in Vancouver I ran in my Hawaiian shirt carrying a pineapple in his honour,' Arry explains. 'I'm sure I looked like quite the eccentric Brit but the Canadians were so supportive and told me my "friend would be proud".'

Jenny and Errol Maginley, from Tring, are another husband and wife who enjoy visiting different parkruns when they are travelling around the UK, Europe and America.

Jenny, 43, a training manager, who has nearly reached the milestone of 500 parkruns, says: 'Most Saturdays Errol and I will attend a parkrun around where we live, or while visiting family and friends. When we're on holiday, we look for parkruns near to where we are staying.' The couple once seized the opportunity to do Hasenheide parkrun in Berlin when they were on holiday in Germany and their flight home was cancelled. 'We got the hotel receptionist to print our barcodes so we could fit in the parkrun before our rescheduled flight,' Jenny recalls. The couple aim to tie parkruns in with trips they are already making, but they did travel to Lucca in Italy specifically for its parkrun. 'We first went there when events were cancelled due to Covid19 and we knew we had to go back to experience doing a parkrun around the city walls,' Jenny said. 'It exceeded my expectations because of the beautiful route with amazing views of the city below.'

Errol, 58, a design engineer agrees this parkrun is 'a rare treat'. He adds of parkrun tourism: 'I love that wherever we go, we can just roll up and meet like-minded runners. Whenever we set off on a parkrun, I find it a satisfying thought that thousands of other parkrunners are all doing the same all over the world.'

One of these parkrunners is John Matthews, 51, from Hertfordshire. parkrun tourism has given him the chance to socialise when travelling the world in his role as a learning technologist, or when travelling for pleasure. He has racked up 627 parkruns, with 182 outside the UK including many in Europe, Australia, Singapore and the USA.

'Throughout my travels, I have found that parkrun always feels the same, despite the differences, which have often been to do with the weather,' he says. John has discovered that in some parts of the world parkruns go ahead with few – if any – marshals and a low number of participants. He liked how at events he attended in Poland, many of the parkrunners introduced themselves to one another with a handshake at the start, while he found Italian parkruns to be 'a bit more racey'. Events in Ireland and New Zealand have been his most memorable for their remote locations and scenery. 'I just love parkrunning on my travels because it helps me see a new place, takes me to places I might otherwise not go to, and meet people I wouldn't otherwise have met,' John says.

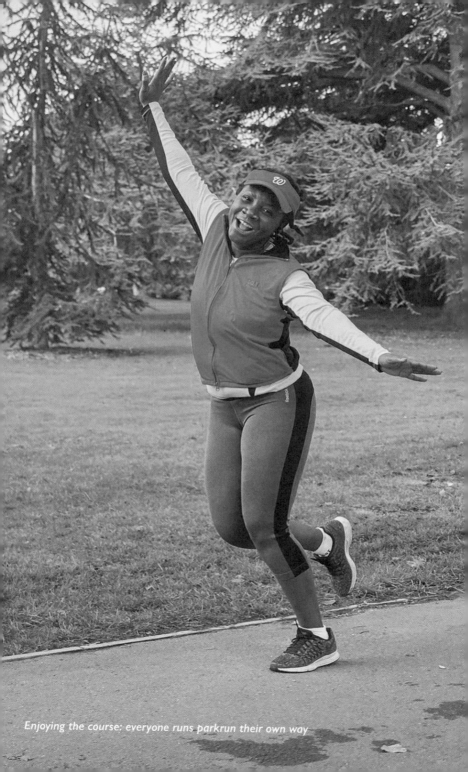
Enjoying the course: everyone runs parkrun their own way

CHAPTER SEVEN

TRAINING, DESTINATION AND CHALLENGE INSPIRATION

The beauty of parkrun is you don't have to be a runner in order to take part. But as outlined in Chapter Four, running can have considerable physical and mental health benefits. So if you do want to get fitter and are able to run, why not give it a go? If you're starting from a very low base of fitness, then following a 'Couch to 5k' plan is a great way to begin and has helped millions of people who thought they could never be a runner do just that. These plans involve walk-running three times a week for up to nine weeks. The run sections gradually increase so that by the end of the schedule, participants should be able to run 5k without stopping. There are various versions of the plan but the most popular in the UK is available as a free app created by Public Health England, in collaboration with the BBC, that can be downloaded onto mobile phones. You can follow the plan solo, or join a running group all following it at the same time where you can meet up to do some of the runs together. Lots of these groups will culminate the plan by getting participants to join in a parkrun when they 'graduate' to becoming a 5k runner. But as you can join in a parkrun and walk the whole way, you don't need to wait until you can run a continuous 5k to join in. You could do any of the walk–runs scheduled in a couch to 5k plan at a parkrun. Also don't be put off by thinking you aren't fast enough once you can run the distance. If you can run for 5k but are finding it takes you 30 minutes or more, you can still join in at a parkrun and you won't be last.

IF YOU FEEL THE NEED FOR SPEED

While you don't have to be fast to do a parkrun, many are moti-vated by trying to lower their time to achieve a PB. So, if this is you, how can you do it? Training consistently will make a big difference. It can take eight weeks for the body to adapt to training, so don't expect to see fitness gains overnight. But if you can stick at it and train three to four times a week, you'll soon notice the difference. If you're new to running, it is important not to do too much, too soon, as this can lead to injury. Follow the couch to 5k plan to begin, and if after that you then want to go further or faster, build up gradually adding five minutes a week to one of your runs, and

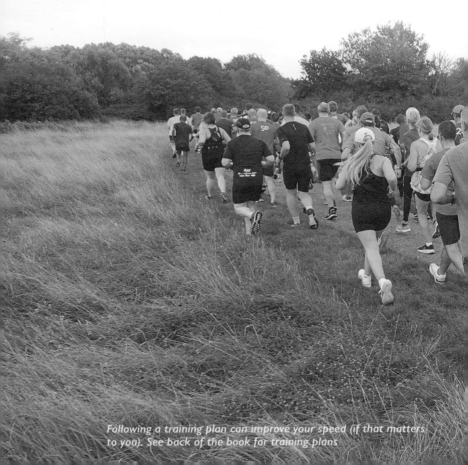

Following a training plan can improve your speed (if that matters to you). See back of the book for training plans

introducing speedwork once a week. This could be in the form of intervals, 'fartleks', tempo runs or hill repetitions. Intervals involve doing a warm up jog for 5-10 minutes, and then doing some time/distance repetitions where you try and run faster than your usual pace, taking a walk/jog recovery in between. For example, you could do 4 x 5 minutes of faster running with 90 seconds walk/jogging in between. On the faster efforts, you should feel like you are working harder than normal. Your heart should be beating faster, and your breathing should be heavier. As these sessions are harder work, you should only do them once a week. You should also aim to do them in a place where you can run the fast efforts without being interrupted to cross a road or having to dodge a lot of people on

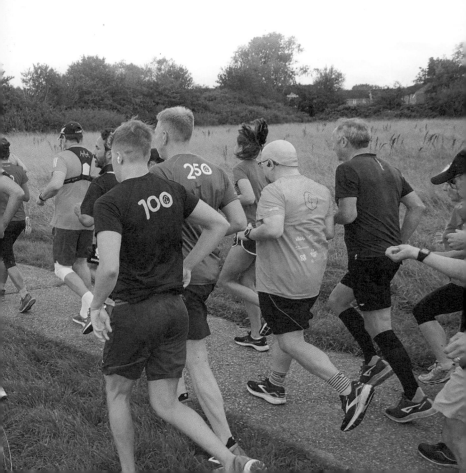

pavements – your local parkrun route could be a good option or an athletics track or paved former railway line.

'Fartleks' are similar to interval sessions but less structured and with more varying paces. For example, if you are doing a 30 minute unstructured fartlek, you can start running easy, then decide when you want to up the pace. You might go faster for a certain amount of time, or till you reach a certain point like the end of a road, and then repeat this, making up when to go faster and slower as you go along. In a structured fartlek, you might run hard for a couple of minutes, and then run at a slightly slower pace (but not easy pace) for a couple of minutes and then repeat. This would be a continuous run rather than breaking it up with the walking/very slow jogging of an interval session. For tempo running, you again want to run at a faster pace than an easy run but not as flat out as a sprint, as the aim is to try and sustain this pace for longer. So you could try 10 minutes easy, 10 minutes at a faster pace, 10 minutes easy. The faster pace should feel 'comfortably uncomfortable'. This is a pace you can then aim to replicate when you are going for a parkrun PB. If you have a target time in mind, you can work out what your pace per mile/k needs to be to achieve it. You can try and run slightly faster

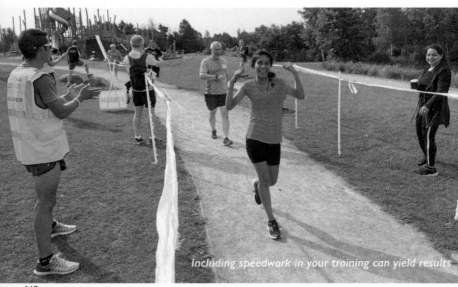

Including speedwork in your training can yield results

than this pace in your intervals, slightly slower than it in tempos, and aim to average this pace in your fartleks. Hill repetitions are another great way to increase your strength, stamina and speed. Again they are hard work so don't do them all the time but about once a month. Run hard up the hill for a set time/distance, jog back down and repeat. These kinds of sessions are often operated by running clubs so joining one is an excellent way to do them with company, and the support of a running coach. Each parkrun event has a list on their website of running club members who regularly participate in that parkrun. This is a good place to start to find a club near you. Some clubs will also do 'volunteer takeovers' where their members will fill the volunteer roles on a specific day, so this is a good opportunity to meet members and find out more about the club.

If you intend to train solo, at the end of the book are some eight-week training plans which incorporate all these elements, and are tailored depending on your target time, to give you some structure and motivation. Follow them and see if you can smash your parkrun PB!

TOP TIPS TO GET FASTER

Include speedwork in your training: See the training plans for a variety of sessions which will help you run faster if you do them regularly.

Do strength work: Doing strength and conditioning will help you stay injury-free and make you a stronger and more efficient runner. You could go to the gym or do your own workout at home using weights or your own body weight for resistance. Pilates and yoga are also excellent ways to improve your strength and flexibility.

Stick with a pacer: Many parkruns have 'pacer' weeks where volunteers will run at a target finishing time. Sticking to the pacer going for the time you want to run can be a big help to keep you going when it starts to feel tough. Hopefully they will have paced it evenly too so you don't go off too fast. If your home parkrun doesn't have set pacers, set your sights on a regular who often seems to run the time you want and try to stay with them.

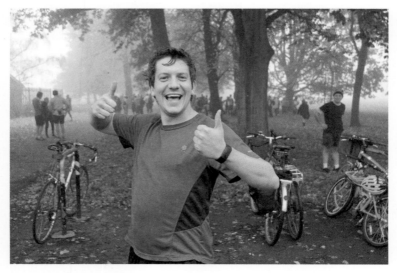

Running a PB is a great feeling

Push yourself: To run faster, it will feel harder and you'll have to push yourself out of your comfort zone. If you are trying your hardest, you won't have the breath to chat to a fellow parkrunner, but you should be able to speak a couple of words like 'thank you marshal!'. Test this out when you are taking part, if you can hold a conversation then you're not at your maximum capacity. Running at your hardest pace can be difficult so you might not want to do this every parkrun if you go every week. Instead, do some easy and then target a week to go faster – as the eight-week training plan recommends.

Pick a fast course: The terrain you are running on makes a big difference to your time. Uneven sections, lots of bends and uphills will slow you down. Check out the list of the fastest UK parkruns in this book. It is worth targeting one of these if you want to see how fast you can really go. Keep in mind the weather will be a factor too. You're unlikely to run your fastest on a very hot day, in humid conditions or when it is freezing cold.

Get super-shoed up: So called super shoes are leading to world records regularly being broken. The shoes have a carbon plate to aid propulsion and are made from foams that improve running economy. Running fast feels easier in these shoes. But note they are expensive and many models aren't that durable so are best saved for PB attempts rather than all runs. Many models don't have great grip too, so are best used on concrete surfaces on dry days.

Join a running club: As part of the club, you'll be able to run with others, benefit from the knowledge and support of their coaches, and do a variety of different sessions which you might struggle for motivation to do alone. Many running club members will parkrun regularly too so you'll get to know even more people at your home event. Check out the 'club list' under the results tab on your local parkrun event page to see which clubs are in your area.

THE FASTEST PARKRUN COURSES IN THE UK

If you want to run a fast parkrun time then the course you run on is a factor. So, how can you find out which is the fastest near you? Checking the average finishing time on the event page gives a rough indication, as does checking the fastest ever male and female times achieved. Note, this information is no longer displayed on the bottom of event homepages but can be found under the 'event history' tab if you order the list by fastest male/female. This also offers an insightful who's who of the elite running scene over the past 20 years, as you'll spot some past and former GB athletes and Olympians on these lists. Another option is to refer to a comprehensive list compiled by Tim Grose, an experienced and speedy runner and the founder and chief statistician of Athletics Data (that operates the Power of 10 and runbritainrankings.com websites). Tim has crunched the numbers to rank the UK parkruns from fastest to slowest using a golf style 'standard scratch score' that takes into account finishing times relative to the course and conditions that day.

His analysis reveals that: 'The fastest courses are typically on a tarmac or similar firm surface, do not have any significant hills, are not too exposed to the wind, and are not too twisty. It can help if there are some other fast runners around you to help with motivation and pacing – but not so many that the route becomes congested and you won't be able to run freely. The fastest UK parkruns tend to be in parks on flat terrain such as Poole parkrun. Then the courses along a seaside promenade, such as Worthing parkrun, can be very fast on a still day but less so on a windy one.'

Tim points out that some courses might be fast because they aren't exactly 5k – and so finishing times should be considered as parkrun PBs and not 5k PBs (and indeed they are runs not races). This is because some UK routes may never have been accurately measured, or on some occasions the start and finish lines may not be placed in the exact positions they are supposed to be by volunteers when setting up that morning. Often alternative courses have to be used too due to the conditions, and these might not have been accurately measured. This is all in the spirit of the original parkrun though, as Paul Sinton-Hewitt discovered the Bushy Park Time Trial route he measured out himself was not quite 5k once he'd called in the professions some time later (so the current Bushy parkrun course is accurate now!).

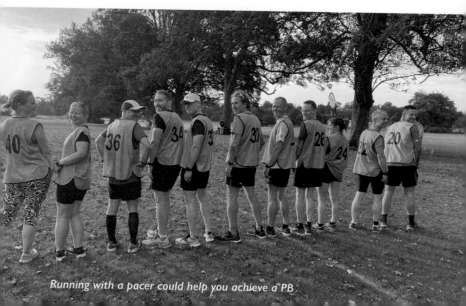

Running with a pacer could help you achieve a PB.

Tim says he hopes fellow parkrunners find his analysis useful, if, like him, they sometimes want to 'race' a parkrun and test their fitness to see how fast they can go. He adds: 'If I am going to be in a certain location, it gives me an indication of what sort of courses to expect from the events I can choose from in that area. Then I can decide which one best suits my inclinations that day, whether I want to test my speed or have more of an offroad challenge. It is good for regular runners to have some variety in their training of tackling slow courses some weeks, as well as fast ones at other times.'

When it comes to the slower courses, Tim says: 'These all tend to be the ones with a soft and uneven surface, such as sand or mud. They may also be very exposed to the wind and/or very hilly. For example, the slowest UK parkrun at Great Yarmouth North Beach has two of these handicaps – it is on sand and tends to be very windy. The next slowest at Whinlatter Forest in the Lake District is very hilly and off-road – you finish a lot higher than you start. Be warned that courses that are all on trail are always going to be slower in the winter and/or after lots of rain because they get muddy and slippery under foot.'

TOP 5 FASTEST COURSES IN THE UK
(BASED ON STATS COMPLIED BY TIM GROSE)

You're most likely to bag a parkrun PB if you can attend one of these speedy events...

5. MUSA Cookstown parkrun, County Tyrone, Northern Ireland:
This course held on the Mid Ulster Sports Complex generates some quick times because it is all on flat, traffic-free tarmac roads for three laps. The average finishing time is 28:27, while the course records are held by Gavin Corey in 14.52 and Grace Carson in 16.46.

4. Hull parkrun, East Yorkshire:
Held in the city's East Park, it is flat as a pancake with just over two laps around a lake on concrete paths. It's hugely popular, with an

average attendance of 532, and an average finishing time of 29:08. The course records are held by Ian Kimpton (14.46) and Becky Briggs (16.36), both athletes who are as speedy over the marathon distance as they are over 5k with PBs there of 2 hours 15 mins and 2 hours 29 respectively.

3. Poole parkrun, Dorset:

This quick course in Poole Park laps a cricket pitch and boating lake offering some pretty views for anyone who is going slow enough to take them in. Perhaps because of the picturesque route and lure of a good time, it is one of the most well-attended in the UK, with 781 participants on average. The highest turnout to date was 1,345, with the average finishing time 27:45. There have been numerous sub 16 minute times achieved here over the years, with the accolade of the fastest ever going to Ben Brown for the men in 14.32 and Melissa Courtney for the women in 15.31.

2. Bromley parkrun, Greater London:

Held in Norman Park, the event runs with a winter course, which is all on tarmac, and a summer route which is partly on grass. The latter doesn't slow times too much on a dry day with the average finishing time throughout the year 28:04. This is another event which is hugely popular with 635 participants on average and a record turnout of 1,051. The fastest ever time recorded was by Michael Skinner with 14.36, with Niamh Bridson Hubbard the fastest female in 16.10.

1. Pegwell Bay parkrun, Kent:

This event is perfect for those looking for both a scenic route and a fast time as it provides coastal views across Pegwell Bay towards Ramsgate. It is flat on compacted gravel paths for two laps. Helping it to the title of the fastest UK parkrun is the fact it is not as well-attended as some of the others in the top five, with an average turnout of 182. This means there is less bunching and bottlenecks at turns (of which there

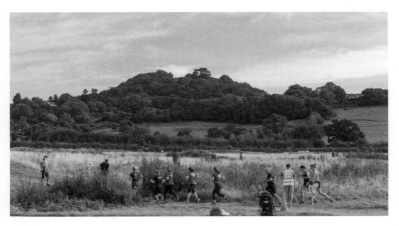

Off-road courses often make for slower times

are actually few on this route too), and more space to run in. Also contributing to it being a PB course for many is that it can be found to be slightly shorter than 5k. However, the course description states it has been 'accurately measured by us with a professional measuring wheel' so the distance covered may depend on the racing line taken. Regardless, it counts as a parkrun PB and the average finishing time is 28:33. The fastest ever times achieved here were by Chris Olley in 14.17 for the men, and Bobby Clay in 16.14 for the women.

TOP 5 SLOWEST PARKRUN COURSES IN THE UK (BASED ON STATS COMPLIED BY TIM GROSE)

Consider these events more of an experience than an opportunity to run your fastest ever parkrun...

5. Mount Edgcumbe, Cornwall:

While this event can't promise speedy PBs, it can deliver amazing views on the South Coast of Plymouth Sound, Cawsand Bay and Drake's Island. These are best seen after climbing up a big hill that contributes to this route being one of the UK's slowest, with parkrunners being encouraged to walk up it so they can take in the spectacular surrounding sights. Times are also slowed down by the course being all off-road on grass and trail paths within Mount Edgcumbe House and Country Park, which also provides additional pretty scenery to take in. The fastest time ever run here by a male was 17.59 by Oliver Paulin, and 20.27 for a female by Annie Arnold, with the average finishing time 31:43.

4. Durlston Country Park, Dorset:

This event in Swanage supplies in stunning scenery what it lacks in speed. On the route, participants go up and down hills along the Jurassic coastline on some steep, narrow paths with views of the English Channel, Bournemouth and Isle of Wight, while passing landmarks such as Durlston Castle and The Great Globe. The fastest times achieved on the trail paths which loops with some tight turns were achieved by Sam Brown Araujo (18.14) and Rebecca Bunting (20.32), while the average finishing time is 35:57.

3. Woolacombe Dunes, Devon:

You know it isn't going to be a flat course when you're warned about a 'dune of doom.' This is one of the sand dunes parkrunners have to tackle on their route along the scenic beach on Devon's North coast. The dunes, soft sand, and exposure to a strong coastal breeze on some occasions all contribute to this being a slow course with an average finishing time of 33:33. The course records are held by Harry Smith in 17.24 for the men, and Amber Gascoigne in 20.22 for the women. While it isn't a PB course, it is a must-visit event for many parkrunners because it offers such a scenic challenge (for more, see the UK Bucket List on page 177).

2. Whinlatter Forest, Cumbria:

This event just outside Keswick in the Lake District has the most elevation in the UK at more than 600 feet. parkrunners start near the bottom of the hill in Whinlatter Forest Park — which the Woodland Trust say is 'England's only true Mountain Forest' — and then climb in a figure of eight on trail paths through the tall pine and ancient oak trees, then past ferns and heather to the finish line. En route they have beautiful views of Grisedale Pike, Skiddaw and Bassenthwaite Lake. Given the hill, the average finishing time is 32:41. The fastest female finishing time of 19.56 is shared by Emma Gould and Sarah McCormack, while Billy Cartwright has the overall record at 17.35.

1. Great Yarmouth North Beach, Norfolk:
This event takes the crown of the slowest in the UK because its two and a half laps are mostly on soft sand and shingle. parkrunners are spared tackling the sand dunes though, as these are out of bounds to protect the resident wildlife. But with its exposed position overlooking the North Sea, strong winds can also be a factor in slowing people down. This is reflected in the records which are a lot slower than the others in the top five. These are held by Robert Chenery in 18.50 and Colleen Mukuya in 21.33, while the average finishing time is 38:36.

See how all the UK parkruns rank in Tim's full list which can be found at **www.thepowerof10.info**

PARKRUN CHALLENGES

While some parkrunners are motivated by going faster, other parkrunners are fans of achieving the various challenges that have developed. The only one officially recognised and rewarded by parkrun is reaching the milestones of 10 (for under 18s), 25, 50, 100, 250, 500, and 1,000 parkruns as a participant or volunteer.

Some parkrunners choose to mark their own milestones such as 200 and 300 to keep themselves motivated between the official totals. Other challenges might involve visiting different locations or finishing in a certain position.

The most popular is the A–Z challenge that involves participating in a parkrun starting with every letter of the alphabet. You can do this within the UK or by travelling abroad. The difficulty of completing the challenge depends on where you live, and how far you are willing or able to travel. For example, there are lots of options around the UK of parkruns beginning with A, B, H and G, but few beginning with J, Q and Y. So for Y, the current options are York parkrun in North Yorkshire, Yarborough Leisure Centre parkrun in Lincoln, and Y Promenâd parkrun, Brecon, in Wales. For a Q, head for Queen's parkruns in Glasgow or Belfast, Queen Elizabeth parkrun in Hampshire, or Quakers Walk parkrun in Devizes, Wiltshire. There are currently no parkruns in the UK starting with the letters Z or X (indeed there aren't any in the world starting with X), so parkrunners have become creative and will accept those with an X in the title such as Exeter Riverside or Exmouth parkrun, both in Devon. For a UK Z, the closest you can get is Sizewell parkrun in Suffolk.

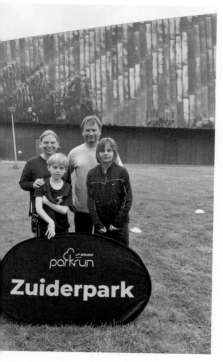

Sara Wroth and her family completing the A–Z Challenge

Completing the challenge minus the X and Z is widely deemed to be acceptable given the lack of options. For those who wish to travel outside the UK, there are numerous Z starting parkruns in countries including Poland and South Africa.

Some people love the alphabet challenge so much, once they have completed it they do it all over again, visiting different letter events to when they completed the first one.

Sara Wroth, 46, a researcher from Hertfordshire, has been parkrunning since 2015 and completed her first Alphabet Challenge in 2024. She started visiting events more strategically after realising she had already collected a few letters from parkruns in her local area. The furthest the mum-of-two travelled for the challenge was to Vejen parkrun in Denmark and Zuiderpark parkrun in the Netherlands, both as part of family holidays. Her longest journey on a Saturday morning in the UK was to Queen Elizabeth parkrun in Hampshire for an elusive 'Q', which was an hour and 20 minute drive for her. Sara said she enjoyed completing the A–Z, along with some other families, because it wasn't about being fast or competitive.

'It gave us an opportunity to spend time with our friends, and with our children, while getting some fresh air and doing something healthy and wholesome,' she says. 'We have been able to explore our local area as well as further afield. I love how every course is different, and every new course is a PB!'

Sara's top tip for anyone doing the Alphabet Challenge is to download the 5K app (more on this to follow) to track your progress and get new venue ideas.

'It will lead you down a rabbit hole to other challenges though!' she warns. 'And don't forget to get a picture of the parkrun name with the event sign!'

As well as the alphabet challenge, other letter challenges are popular, such as doing a parkrun in every letter of your name or with every letter of 'parkrun'. Meanwhile, there are some number challenges. So people might try to form a number sequence using the event number of the parkrun they attend that day.

Trying to attain some famous number sequences is discouraged by parkrun HQ as it can lead to people turning up en masse at a certain event, such as an inaugural parkrun because they want a number 'one'.

Large numbers suddenly turning up can put a strain on volunteers. parkrun used to publish a league table of who had attended the most inaugural events but it was taken down to discourage such surges. Its Global Chief Operating Officer Tom Williams published an open letter to parkrun tourists in 2023 appealing to them to avoid challenges that encourage attendance at a particular event on a specific day. He wrote that it poses a danger – not only to participants and volunteers that day but also to the future of that event – because 'it places teams under unreasonable levels of pressure whilst increasing a number of risks associated with event delivery.'

This is why parkrun also abolished allowing parkruns in the UK to start at different times of the morning on New Year's Day, as people were rushing to get to one start at 9am and then another at 10am in order to achieve a 'New Year's Day Double'. Tom wrote that this challenge resulted in 'operational challenges to a level that we could not mitigate safely, which resulted in us moving to a position where people could only record one parkrun on any one day.'

THERE'S AN APP FOR THAT

While you can use your official parkrun profile linked to your barcode to track how many parkruns you have done and where, it isn't able to tell you how you are working towards the various challenges that have become popular. So, many parkrunners use unofficial apps to track challenges and get new ideas. One of the most popular is called '5k'. The app is not endorsed or supported by parkrun but users can scan their barcode into it and retrieve a record of all the parkruns they have done. The app then automatically logs which challenges have been completed already, with a percentage of how far a person has to go to complete others. The app also provides event details on courses where people can view stats on attendance, and read reviews from other app users who have been to the event. The map search function is particularly useful in helping parkrun tourists find nearby events when they are travelling.

The app was started by Mike Clayton, 33, who is himself a keen parkrunner who has attended more than 214 at nearly 80 different locations. He said: 'What has always kept me coming back to parkrun is that it isn't just a run. I've made a fair few

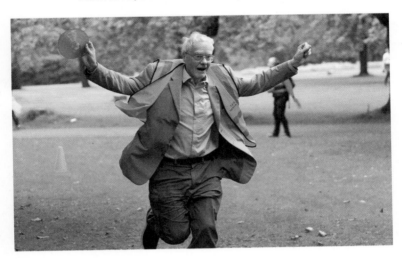

Volunteering at parkrun is fun

friends at my home event so the highlight is breakfast at the cafe afterwards. I also enjoy touring to new events with friends and seeing new places. The idea for the 5k app came about during a conversation with some friends at one of our post parkrun cafe catch-ups in 2019. We realised that there was no parkrun app and at the time the parkrun website was not mobile friendly, so trying to look up your results on a phone screen was not easy. As I'm a software engineer, somebody suggested that I try to make an app. I initially launched it in 2019 for Android and then several months later for iOS.'

Since then a couple of hundred thousand parkrunners have downloaded 5k, despite it never having been advertised. The app includes many of the most popular challenges like the Alphabet and Compass Club (attending a parkrun beginning North, East, South and West.)

The parkrun community help shape the app by making suggestions. Mike says: 'Just like parkrun, I always intend to keep this app free for people to download and use.'

POPULAR PARKRUN CHALLENGES

Alphabet AKA Alphabeteer or A-Z Challenge: Attend a parkrun starting with every letter of the alphabet.

Cowell Club: Attend 100 different parkrun locations. This challenge is named after the first person who achieved this. You can gain just a 'Cow' for reaching 50 locations.

Compass club: Attend a parkrun beginning with the four letters of the compass points – North, East, South and West.

County Challenge: Attend every parkrun in a certain UK county eg Norfolk.

Date bingo: Attend a parkrun on every day in a year, this will take multiple years to complete.

Double-ton: Attend 200 parkruns at the same location.

Festive Double: Attend a parkrun on Christmas Day and New Year's Day in the same festive season.

Groundhog Day: Finish with the same time, at the same location, at consecutive parkruns.

Jetsetter: Attend a parkrun in five different countries.

LonDONE: Visit every parkrun in the capital.

Monthly: Attend a parkrun in every month of the year.

NENDY Quest: NENDY stands for 'Nearest Event Not Done Yet', which is the closest event to your current location which you haven't attended. It can be never-ending if a new parkrun pops up close to where you live, and the list will keep refreshing with your next nearest NENDY once you've ticked off your closest one.

Position bingo: Get every finishing position from 1-99. You don't need to be fast to complete this one, as 114, 214 etc still counts as position 14.

UK Tourist: Attend 20 different parkruns in the UK.

Tourist Streak: Attend five different parkrun locations in a row.

Volunteer Bingo: Volunteer in every role available.

Volunteer Streak: Volunteer at five different parkrun locations in a row.

Volunteer Tourist: Volunteer at 10 different parkrun locations.

Ultimate World Tourist: Visit a parkrun in every country where there is one.

UK PARKRUN BUCKET LIST:
10 OF THE BEST PARKRUNS IN THE UK

Just like with the global bucket list, there are so many that could have made this top 10. These parkruns in England, Northern Ireland, Scotland and Wales all have unique features and spectacular scenery. They are in areas already popular with tourists so could be tied in with a holiday...

1. FOUNTAINS ABBEY PARKRUN, NORTH YORKSHIRE:

The scenery is spectacular at this World Heritage site, set in a secluded valley and deer park. Participants pass the ruins of Fountains Abbey, the largest monastic ruins in the country. The Abbey was founded in 1132 by 13 Benedictine monks from St Mary's in York but fell into disrepair following the Dissolution of the Monasteries ordered by Henry VIII. It links up with the elegant Studley Royal Water Garden, a series of romantically designed picturesque ponds, statues and follies that is considered to be one of the finest

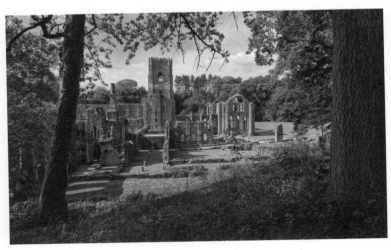

The ruins of Fountains Abbey. (Wikimedia Commons)

examples of a Georgian water garden in England, created by John Aislabie in 1718. Both sites are now owned by the National Trust. As if that isn't enough, parkrunners also get to amble past the flowing River Skell and see wildlife such as deer, woodpeckers and swans. On average 435 parkrunners attend each week, in an average time of 29:13. Many say it is the most beautiful parkrun they have ever done.

2. BUSHY PARKRUN, WEST LONDON:

Many parkrunners are keen to make the 'pilgrimage' to Bushy to see where it all started. Given it is in Teddington, an area of London well-populated with runners, attendance is always high regardless of the influx of tourists who want to retread the steps of the parkrun pioneers. On average it attracts a gigantic 1,381 participants. The record attendance at the time of publication was 2,545. Those who are used to running at small events will be amazed by the stampede of runners at the start, and the slick organisation of the

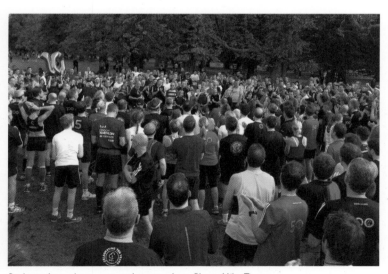

Bushy parkrun always attracts large numbers. Photo: Mike Tivnen

volunteers who cope admirably with the swarm of finishers. They have a special dual (sometimes triple) funnel system to ensure the finishing tokens are all handed out in the correct order. Not only is Bushy worth visiting because it is the first event and such a large parkrun to be part of, it is also a beautiful park to run in. It is home to ancient trees, herds of deer and fountains including the 17th century Diana Fountain of the goddess of the hunt, which is by the parkrun start. The route is flat for those hunting a PB, with an average finish time of 27:42. The historic royal palace of Hampton Court is also next door and the River Thames.

3. SEVERN BRIDGE PARKRUN, MONMOUTHSHIRE, WALES:

This parkrun is unique because the course is both in Wales AND England. Starting in Monmouthshire, Wales, parkrunners run up to and over the famous long suspension bridge with amazing views of the Severn Estuary below (as long as it isn't a foggy day!). Before turning back, they cross the national border into the English counties of Gloucestershire and Avon. Once back in Wales, they run down from the bridge to finish in a brightly painted underpass. The route is predominantly flat on a wide concrete path beside the M48, whose drivers sometimes honk their horns to cheer on the runners. On average 237 attend with an average finish time of 29:04.

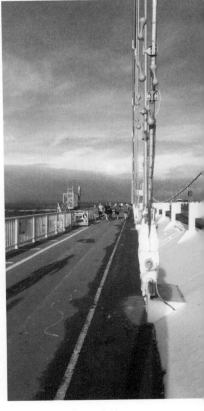

parkrunners on Severn Bridge
© Marco Paganuzzi

4. EDEN PROJECT PARKRUN, CORNWALL:

parkrunners get free entry (at the time of the event only) to one of the UK's top tourist attractions, a collection of plants from around the world, which celebrates the natural world. parkrunners pass by the famous giant biomes as they zig-zag around the venue, and then have stunning views of them as they climb hills and loop back down again. Despite the undulating path and twists and turns, the average time is 29:40 for the 314 finishers on average, many of whom combined their run with a holiday in Cornwall.

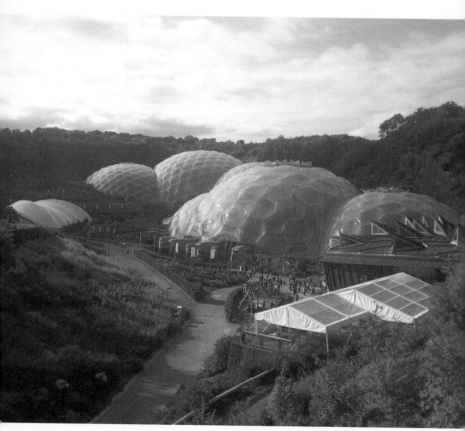

The spectacular biomes at The Eden Project in Cornwall (Wikimedia Commons)

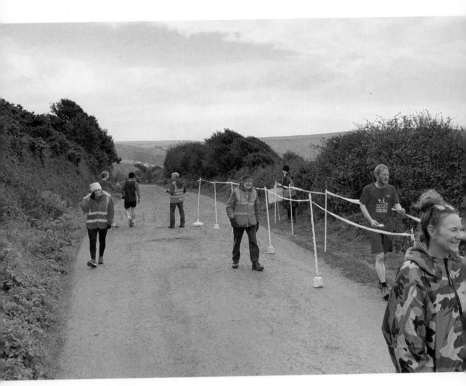

parkrun amid hills and beautiful scenery © aparkrunner/Flikr

5. WOOLACOMBE DUNES PARKRUN, DEVON:

Another parkrun that regularly attracts holidaymakers in the area, with an average turn out of 144. It is one of the slowest parkruns in the UK, with an average finishing time of 33:33, because it is partly run on a sandy beach and over some tricky sand dunes. Many make the visit to take on the 'Dune of Doom' on the course, while the coastal weather can be an extra challenge if it is wet and windy. On a calm and sunny day though, it is idyllic. So while it is not one to visit for a PB, you can test your stamina while taking in the surrounding scenery and wildlife of this event held on National Trust land within an Area of Outstanding Beauty.

6. PORTRUSH PARKRUN, NORTHERN IRELAND:

While Portrush wasn't the first event to start in Northern Ireland (that was Belfast's Waterworks parkrun in 2010), when it was launched in 2012 Portrush was the very first parkrun held entirely on a beach. It goes out and back along the sand of East Strand Beach, providing jaw-dropping views of the rocky coastline, with the Skerries Islands on the horizon out to sea. While running on the

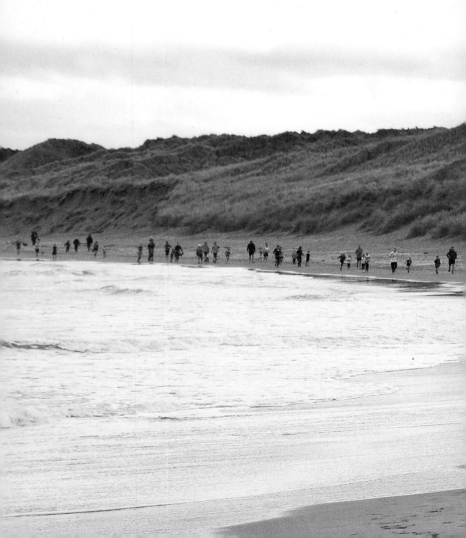

soft sand can be slow-going and exposed to winds off the Atlantic ocean, when the tide has recently been in it makes the sand firmer to give an average finishing time of 29:47 for the 217 finishers. In warmer months, many of these enjoy a dip in the water afterwards. Around the corner from the route in Antrim is the World Heritage Site of Giant's Causeway which is worth a visit after the parkrun to see the iconic basalt columns formed following a volcanic eruption millions of years ago.

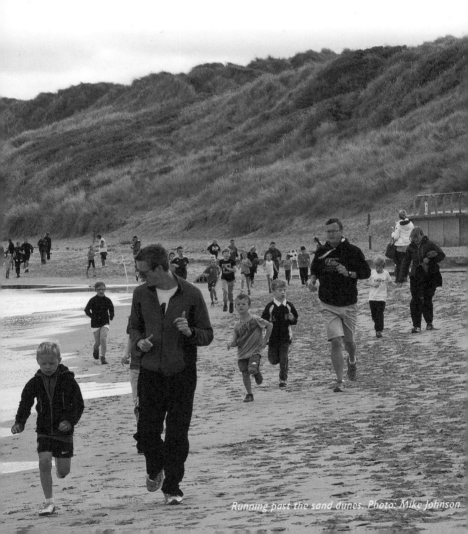

Running past the sand dunes. Photo: Mike Johnson

7. SOMERDALE PAVILION PARKRUN, SOMERSET:

You might get dizzy at this event, also known as the 'curly wurly one'. This is because the route winds around and around a spiral cut into the grass on the Shamcross Cyclocross course, creating a bonkers course map that looks like it has been scribbled by a toddler. As this event is held all on grass on private land in Bristol that is prone to flooding, it sometimes has to be cancelled at short notice. On average there are 151 runners a week with an average finishing time of 29:14. Take yourself for a spin there if you can.

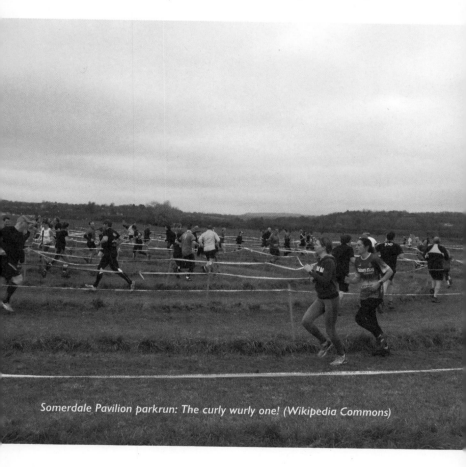

Somerdale Pavilion parkrun: The curly wurly one! (Wikipedia Commons)

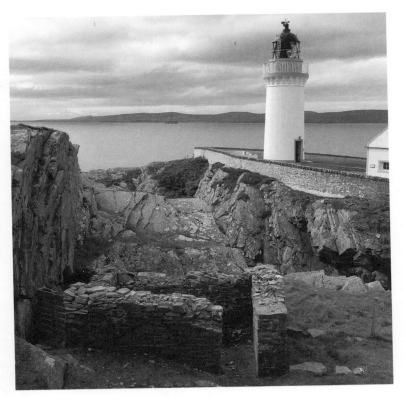

Bressay lighthouse. Photo: Rob Farrow, Creative Commons

8. BRESSAY PARKRUN, SHETLAND ISLANDS:

This is the most northerly parkrun in the UK but is beaten in the world northerly rankings by a few in Scandinavia. As it is such a remote rural location with a population of 360, getting there is part of the adventure and the event might be cancelled if the inter-island Saturday ferry isn't running. The scenic out and back route is on public roads with views of the sea and unspoilt countryside. parkrunners are advised to keep left at all times in case any of the islanders are out in their cars after the 9.30am start. The average attendance since the event launch in 2018 is 44, with an average finishing time of 32:04.

9. HOLYROOD PARKRUN, EDINBURGH:

For sweeping views of Scotland's capital city, head to this event in Holyrood park. It loops for one big lap on a closed road, starting next to the serene swan covered St Margaret's Loch. It then climbs steeply up part of Arthur's Seat for 1.5k, which is worth the effort for the views. These can be appreciated as the route flattens out before a steep descent back down where parkrunners again see the sights of the City below. Despite the rugged surrounding terrain and tough uphill, the average time is quicker than the national average at 28:48 because it is all on tarmac, and what goes up must come down. It is regularly well-attended with 428 parkrunners on average and a start time of 9.30am.

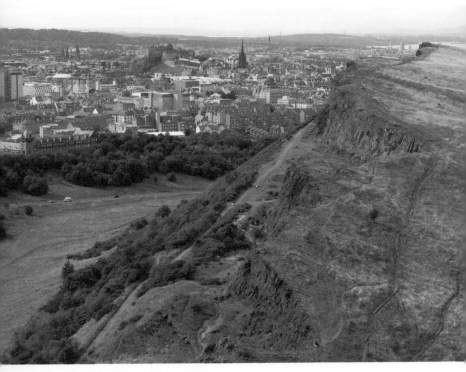

Holyrood parkrun offers spectacular views of Edinburgh around Arthur's Seat (© Spencer Means/Flikr)

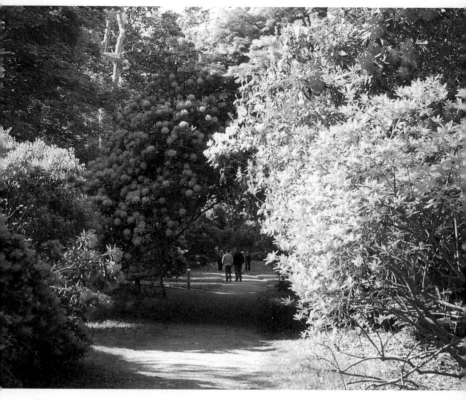

Sheringham parkrun, surrounded by rhododendrons in spring. Photo: Chris Wood, Creative Commons

10. SHERINGHAM PARKRUN, NORFOLK:

Another event held on a National Trust site of Sheringham Park. The route passes through a beautiful pine forest which is abundant with blossoming rhododendrons in the Spring. One section at the edge of the forest offers panoramic views of the North sea off the North Norfolk coast with the Weybourne windmill in view, and you might see a steam train chuff past along the nearby heritage 'Poppy' Line between Sheringham and Holt. The commonly held belief that Norfolk is flat is debunked here as the route is undulating with parkrunners having to climb up a hill to reach the finish, making the average finishing time 30:31 for the 174 attendees.

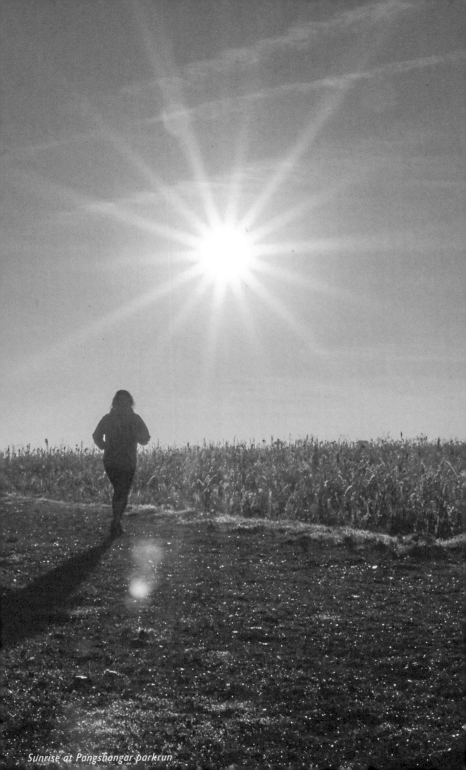

Sunrise at Pangshangar parkrun

CHAPTER EIGHT:
THE FUTURE

PARKRUN'S FIVE YEAR PLAN

In 2023, parkrun published its five-year global strategy, outlining how it intends to grow and develop. Just as Paul Sinton-Hewitt envisioned when he set up the first event, the goal remains to minimise barriers to participation so more people can gain health and happiness from being active outdoors, while surrounded by nature and socialising with other people. Attracting more participants means setting up new venues around the world and encouraging more people to attend existing events. To support this expansion, the 'parkrun world' has been divided into four regions: America; APAC (Asia Pacific); EMEA (Europe, Middle East and Africa); and the UK. Each region is responsible for growing parkrun sustainably across its territory. The idea is to alleviate some of the pressure on global parkrun HQ and give each of the regions more autonomy. To fund this expansion, parkrun says it 'must continue to increase revenue and ensure financial sustainability by consolidating existing income streams, driving efficiencies, improving resources and continuing to explore new opportunities across retail, commercial partnerships, public fundraising and public grants.' If the plan is a success, parkrun hopes to double both the number of events and weekly participants around the world, respectively from 2,200 to 4,400, and from 250,000 to 500,000 by 2028.

POTENTIAL NEW PARKRUN PLACES

Many of the new events and participants will come from areas of the world where few, or no parkruns, are offered, or where event participation

DID YOU KNOW?
When starting parkrun, Paul Sinton-Hewitt said it was his dream that there might one day be a parkrun in every town in the world.

is currently low. Russ Jefferys, the chief executive, says parkrun has received numerous requests to set up new events in various parts of the world, and it is now in a position to start exploring these new venues and territories further. He said: 'Now we have more of a strategy and resources, we can start taking some of those requests forward. We are lucky in that there are active requests for parkruns in dozens of countries worldwide including

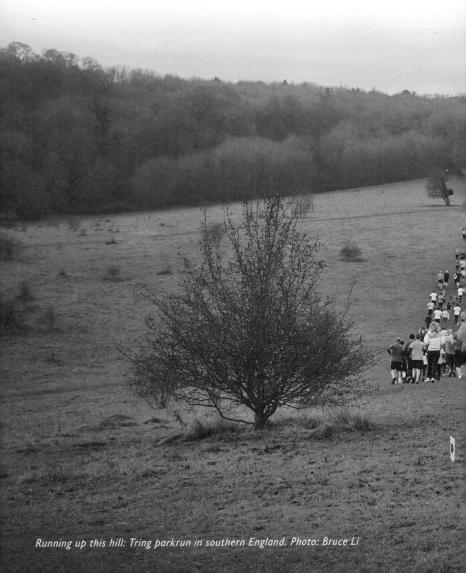

Running up this hill: Tring parkrun in southern England. Photo: Bruce Li

Portugal, Belgium, Switzerland and Spain. Then in Africa, we have parkruns in three countries but it is a huge continent and there are lots of opportunities and interest there. In particular, we are looking at East Africa and we have had teams visit Uganda. In central and South America and parts of Asia we have no presence, so there could be some movement on that over the next few years.'

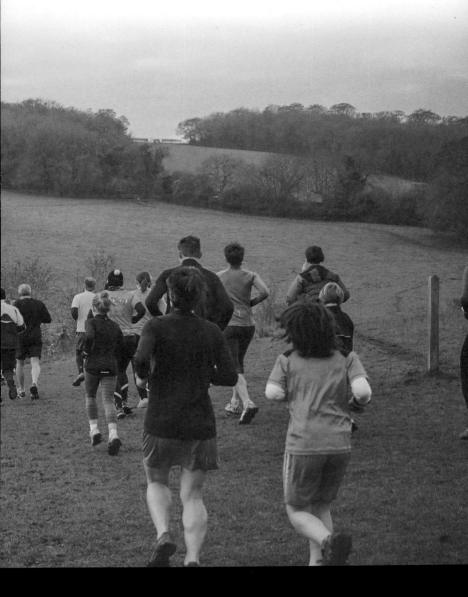

Jefferys admits there are 'some obvious gaps' around the world where parkruns could be held and be successful, but the plan is to 'focus on where there is demand, or where we think there can be great impact.' He explained: 'We always take the view that we don't want parkrun to be imposed on a local community, it needs to be wanted and delivered by that local community. So we would need to raise awareness of what parkrun is in any given country or location before thinking about starting one.'

Meanwhile, there are also plans to increase the number of junior parkruns and expand existing ones to include more children. In the UK, plans are afoot to make this possible thanks to the London Marathon Foundation (LMF) giving £1.19 million to be spent on getting an additional 300,000 children active in the next three years, particularly in disadvantaged communities.

WHO ISN'T PARKRUNNING AND WHY?

In order to get more weekly participants, parkrun must understand and break down barriers to attendance. Research conducted on parkrun participation in Australia, published in 2013 and 2018, found at individual level, higher attendance has 'been associated with being married/partnered, having lower levels of education, and being a non-runner at registration.' In 2022, parkrun conducted a survey in the UK, Ireland and Australia to find out why a great number of those who register for a barcode never actually attend, or only attend once. The results revealed that: for 20 percent the start time was inconvenient; 13 per cent felt too unfit to take part; 12 per cent were ruled out by injury/illness; another 12 per cent didn't have time; and 10 percent had childcare obligations. Then nine per cent were put off because they didn't know what to expect; another nine per cent didn't want to intend alone; while smaller numbers said

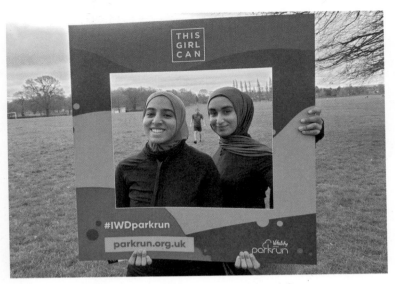

parkrun staged a 'This Girl Can' campaign on International Women's Day to encourage more women and girls to take part

they felt 5k was too far, or they were concerned about running in public. More women than men were likely not to attend because of a perceived lack of fitness. Steps have been taken to counter this by encouraging more people to attend as walkers instead of runners, and making the events seem less intimidatingly competitive by removing the data on fastest ever recorded times. The authors of the survey pointed out that changing the start time in the future is unlikely to be helpful in boosting numbers, since there will never be a time convenient for everyone. To overcome the childcare issues, the authors recommended further promotion on how parkrun is a family-friendly event, where children can join in with their parents by running, walking or volunteering, or babies and young children can be pushed in running buggies.

Encouraging more people from deprived and non-white ethnic backgrounds to join in is another way to increase participation. While accurate stats on the ethnicity of all parkrunners can't be obtained because people do not have to reveal this upon registration, a survey carried out in 2018 on UK parkrunners with

60,694 respondents found 96.1 per cent of them were white. The survey also found that just 11.5 percent of the parkrunners questioned come from deprived communities. Separate research studies on parkruns in England in 2018 found lower participation rates in areas with higher ethnic density and lower socioeconomic status.

parkrun is considering what it can do to increase participation. Russ Jefferys said: 'Largely parkrun has grown through word of mouth, and that tends to stay contained within demographics. We need to understand with better data exactly who is participating. We need to do more with the GP practices, have more outreach in different communities and essentially try to understand what the local needs and barriers are. We hope to work with other

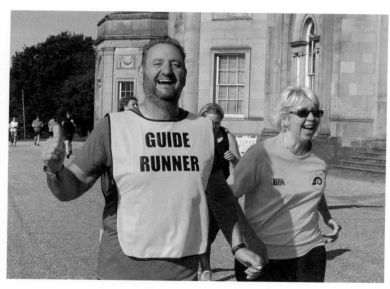

Guide runners help people with sight difficulties participate

organisations to do this. Why is it that we might have an event in an area that is predominantly non-white but the parkrun attendance is predominantly white? What can we do to effect change there?'

He added: 'Essentially, I think it is about working with local people and understanding local conditions and coming up with solutions.'

However he knows that parkrun won't be the solution for everyone. 'There will be fundamental structural barriers in place that mean some people can't take part on a Saturday morning for whatever reason,' he said. 'That is fine, we just want to make sure we are doing our bit to reach as many people as possible – particularly those who would benefit the most.'

REMOVING 'OFF-PUTTING STATS'

At the start of 2024, parkrun removed all the lists of the fastest 500 runners, first finishers, sub 20/17 minute runners and course and age category records from its websites. Sharing the reasons behind the move in a statement, parkrun's head of communications, Kirsty Woodbridge, said research with its global working group had found this data could be 'off-putting' to potential new parkrunners. By prominently displaying the quickest times, it seemed it was scaring off people who didn't want to be competitive, and who thought they could only join in if they could run fast. A separate study carried out in Australia analysing the growth of parkrun events came to a similar conclusion. It found: 'parkruns with a less competitive social milieu may have more rapid dissemination.' Russ explains that the stat removal 'was a small thing we did to chip away at the idea that parkrun is a race. Previously, we were saying "parkrun is not a race" but then sharing information that contradicted that statement.'

Removing the stats didn't go down well with all parkrunners, especially those who used to enjoy going for age graded records, racking up first finishes, or seeing the course records at a glance to determine how challenging a route might be.

One of them, Rich Harrison, 54, a regular at parkruns in East Yorkshire and North Lincolnshire, said: 'As someone who has held age group category records in the past – and had hoped to in the future – taking them away has given me one less thing to aim for. I loved going for these as it inspired me to keep racing and training as I age.' He knew a number of elderly runners who enjoyed going around different parkruns trying to gain age category records, and this element was lost to them now. He said he will still be motivated to get a high age-grading when he takes part but 'taking away some of the stats that made parkrun such a huge success has saddened me greatly.'

Gavin Caney, who was once the course record holder at Downham Market Academy parkrun in Norfolk with a time of 16.45, felt that parkrun had 'created an environment of competition and racing until it no longer suited them'.

'If parkrun is truly for all, you cannot erase the one thing that many people often enjoyed about it – racing against others and trying to set new records,' he said. 'parkrun celebrates so much but no longer those who sometimes take it seriously.' Mary Taylor felt so strongly about it, she started an online petition urging parkrun to 'bring back the stats', which was signed by thousands of people. She wrote on change.org: 'The removal of statistics from parkrun has left a void in the hearts of many participants. These stats are not just numbers; they represent personal milestones and progress that inspire runners of all abilities to push their limits. Statistics have always been an integral part of parkrun. They provide a tangible measure of improvement and motivate participants to keep striving for better results.'

At parkrun, chief executive Russ Jefferys doubled down on its decision, publishing an open letter explaining why the changes were staying. 'We have a sharp, unwavering focus on removing the barriers to participation which persist for many people, especially for those whom physical activity may not be the norm, those who may never engage with traditional "sports", or be able to afford gyms or other subscriptions, or find any inclusive and welcoming spaces for move-ment… The fear of finishing last, of being the "slowest", of not being

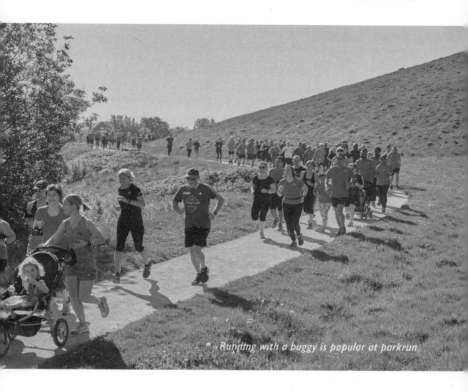

Running with a buggy is popular at parkrun.

celebrated, of not being as good as everyone else, or not even able to finish at all. None of these things should be a barrier to joining parkrun, but it certainly wasn't helpful that we were providing prominent links to a considerable amount of data from our home pages that was clearly performance related,' he wrote.

There was much speculation that parkrun's decision to stop the course records being so prominently displayed, and to remove the gender age category records completely, was because of controversy over trans-gender athletes holding some of these records. Some felt it wasn't fair that a parkrunner born a man could compete in the female category after transitioning, as they still might have a biological advantage over those born female. Implying in his open letter that this did not influence parkrun's decision, Jefferys wrote: 'I have never advocated taking the easy option if it isn't the right thing to do. In this instance, it was obvious we needed to modify our websites if we were to be true to our mission and values. It is as simple as that. There is no hidden agenda at play.'

Many parkrunners welcomed the change to remove the stats.

Claire Davis, who has Multiple Sclerosis and has clocked up 66 parkruns at 18 locations, started parkrunning after completing the Couch to 5k plan and would happily jog at the back. She was surprised when she saw how seriously people at the front were taking it when she volunteered as a barcode scanner. 'I saw the first two finishers pushing themselves over the finish line and they were practically dead, huffing and puffing like crazy. It was incredibly puzzling for me and I just couldn't get my head around it,' she recalls. 'It had never even crossed my mind before then that people would treat it as a race. It is all about enjoyment and fun for me. And just getting there can be a challenge as I can often feel fatigued because I have MS, plus I need to organise childcare for my two children. This is why I find targeting milestones more motivating than going for times. Personally, I'm glad the records are gone as now runners at the front might take it less seriously.'

Others, like Ruth Crowther, who has been a parkrunner since 2012, say the stat removal hasn't made any difference to their enjoyment. 'I don't care about the stats. I just love the community aspect,' she says. 'I used to race it against my own times and realised I wasn't really enjoying it so I changed to thinking it was just a social run at a slower pace. My other training runs are usually solo and I take part in races so it's nice just to run with others on a Saturday morning in a non-race environment.' Ruth, who records her parkrun time on her watch, goes as far as to say she wouldn't even mind if there were no published results at all.

Speaking of the future, Jefferys said he 'can't imagine a time where we don't time parkruns as it pretty integral'. For those who do love to know how they fared, parkrun continues to send an email after each event to everyone who scanned their personal barcode with their finishing time, position and age grading. The full set of results continue to be available to view each week on each event page, showing finishing order, those who ran PBs, and what everyone's age grading was. You can reorder the results to show who had the best age grading that day, and who has done the most total parkruns by changing the sorting order via a box at the top of the results, with additional information provided switching from the 'compact' to 'detailed' view. And for those who want more stats, each event page now has an 'event history' section where you can see who the first male and first female finisher was each week with their time. You can also see how many attended and how many volunteered. The list is shown automatically chronologically from the most recent week down to the very first event. You can change the view to list the fastest recorded male or fastest recorded female finishing times – which means you can still find out the course records if you really want to. The course records, and all age category records for each event are also currently still available via unofficial sources such as the '5k' app.

DISCOURAGING PARKRUN TOURISM?

Another stat change made at the start of 2024 was to remove lists on parkrun websites celebrating who had participated in the most events. Russ said this decision was not taken because parkrun is 'anti-tourism or anti-wanting people to do a challenge'. But because this information had become 'a bit outdated' and wasn't inclusive of celebrating all parkrunners because 'if you are starting your parkrun journey today, there is no hope of you appearing on those pages.' He added that the list is also a bit 'meaningless' given the majority of parkrunners only go to their home event.

parkrun is concerned about the environmental impact too. When it comes to visiting venues, parkrun encourages people to get there with the lowest carbon footprint possible. Each event website has the following message on its course information page: 'Please, wherever possible walk, jog, cycle or use public transport when attending the event. If you do have to drive, please consider car-sharing to reduce

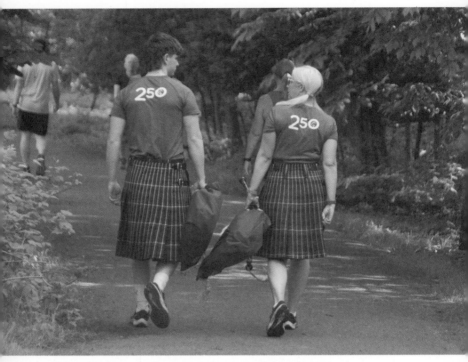

Racking up parkruns at various venues is why some people love taking part

our impact on both the environment and other park users.' Jefferys, however, says it is important that people have the 'individual freedom' to decide where they will parkrun and how they will get there as 'people find lots of different reasons to enjoy parkrun and different motivations. It is not for us to be too prescriptive.'

THE FUTURE OF RESULTS

While the intention remains for parkruns always to be timed, Russ Jefferys revealed the nature of how the results are shared publicly could change in the future. He said: 'There is a question about how much personal data we make publicly available for data security, privacy, scalability etc. When parkrun started with a handful of events, the amount of data we were sharing was very small. Now with thousands of events around the world and continued growth, there is a huge amount of publicly available data. We have had feedback from some people who would prefer an anonymous profile, or for their parkrunning to be private.'

People who don't currently want to appear in the results can do so by ducking out of the finish funnel and not getting a token – although this then doesn't give parkrun an accurate reflection of the number who attended a particular event that day. Another current option for people to remain anonymous is to take a finishing token and get it scanned but then not have their personal barcode scanned. The flaw with this is they don't get their official time and the run won't be counted towards their milestones.

While there is currently no way for people to participate anonymously while still gaining an official time and participation credit, the idea is under consideration. parkrun is considering developing more private profiles, like the running app Strava. And so, you could choose whether to share your activities publicly, or just keep them to yourself.

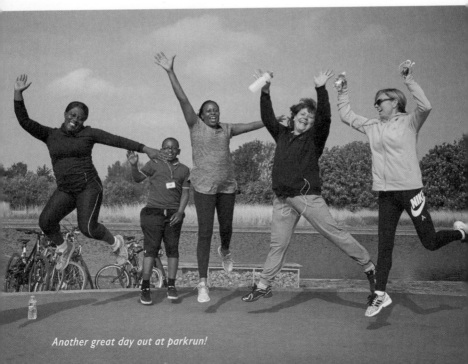

Another great day out at parkrun!

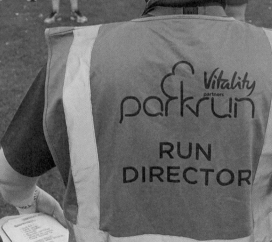

Briefing runners at Reading parkrun in England

CHAPTER NINE

HOW TO SET UP YOUR OWN PARKRUN

If you're keen to set up a parkrun in your area, fill in a form on parkrun's website with the proposed venue. You will receive help and support from parkrun HQ and its regional ambassadors to see if the new parkrun can be brought to life. parkrun chief executive Russ Jefferys said the first step should be ensuring there is a core team ready and willing to deliver the event each week so there is a 'shared responsibility and ownership for the event'. As shown at the very first parkrun with four volunteers, Paul Sinton-Hewitt couldn't do it alone, and he needed lots of help and support as the event grew. Each new event needs a dedicated team to ensure it can keep going. Getting the permission of the landowner is paramount. Current events are held on land that might belong to, for example a local council, the National Trust, the Woodland Trust or an individual. Another key consideration is the impact introducing a parkrun would have on the surrounding community. This means not only being able to have a course that is safe for people to run on and access in potentially large numbers, but in doing so in a way that doesn't negatively impact non-parkrun users of the area. The impact on the environment is a big factor too. Does the venue have decent public transport links? Is the site an area of special historic or ecological interest that might need to be protected? This will not necessarily rule out an event being held there. As seen throughout this Guide, parkrun events are held in conservation areas such as World Heritage Sites, National Parks or Sites of Special Scientific Interest. What it does mean is that extra considerations should be undertaken to protect the precious habitats and buildings. While encouraging people to attend 'under their own steam' or via public transport, parkrun acknowledges that for many, driving will be the only option so each new event needs to have suitable and safe parking. This is both for the safety of participants and to reduce the impact on the surrounding areas, so that local residents are not blocked into their houses by parkrunners parking across their driveways, or causing traffic jams as they come and go.

COURSE CONSIDERATIONS

parkrun has a number of recommendations for an ideal course. Placing the start and finish in the same location, or close together, is preferred to an A to B route. This is so the volunteers don't have to move equipment further and the start and finish teams will be in proximity to enhance the social element. When few volunteers are available, it also makes it easier for multiple roles to be undertaken by one person. The start and finish areas should have enough space to allow parkrunners to congregate without getting in the way of other park users. Entering a narrow path or sharp turn should be avoided at the start of the course, so participants don't have bottle-necks or run into one another. Also, downhills should be avoided at the start or finish as these naturally make people run faster which is more likely to cause issues when people are close together at the start, or sprinting into the finish funnel at the end.

Meanwhile, parkrun points out: 'Whilst it can be natural to think that meandering one-lap courses that take in as many of the local sights and sounds as possible would be far more attractive to parkrunners, our experience tells us that this isn't the case... Multi-lap courses are significantly easier to cover with volunteers.' Additionally it is recommended that courses do not cross roads that are open to the public or cross car parks (ironically the first time trial route in Bushy Park did this). Furthermore, routes should not cross cattle grids, go over fencing or down steps, and ideally shouldn't pass through gates (if they do a marshal will be needed to hold the gate open throughout the event). When considering a route, it needs to be able to accommodate at least 150 participants, with an awareness that numbers could hugely increase on days of special interest (such as Christmas Day) or if the event rapidly gains in popularity. There needs to be space for runners to be overtaken on lapped routes, and to avoid collisions on out and back paths. It also needs to be not too complicated or difficult to follow, particularly in light of the fact marshals may not always be available. Thus parkrun states that it should only take a couple of lines to describe a route on a course description. If not, it probably needs to be simplified.

While many parkruns take place on hillsides, beaches and on coastal paths, this needs to be risk assessed to ensure there are no steep drops or dangerously uneven terrain. It is useful for venues to have an alternative course option·for times when the weather might create issues for an event going ahead, for example, if a path is icy or flooded. Alternative courses should be slightly longer so people don't set PBs they can't then attain again on the usual 5k course.

junior parkruns can be held on the same sites as parkruns but parkrun recommends they are led by different teams so the responsibility each week for both isn't falling on the same people. Using an existing site for a junior parkrun is useful as then there is already a relationship established with the landowner. However, junior parkruns can also explore new, smaller venues, as the route needs to only cover 2k. Some are held within the grounds of schools or simply lap playing fields in a park.

'HOW WE SET UP THRIVING PARKRUNS'

Kate Tettmar, 53, a Senior Clinical Scientist from Hertfordshire, was part of the core team who set up Heartwood Forest parkrun in Sandridge in 2017. Kate already had experience as part of the core team at another local event – St Albans parkrun – and they were keen for another in the area to help alleviate numbers, which were often close to 500. Kate recalls: 'We had some funding from

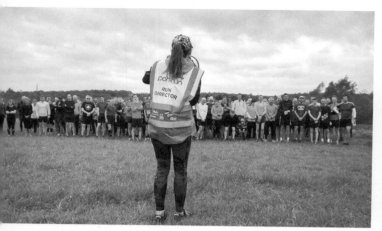
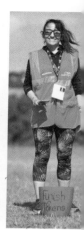

Jersey Farm Event Director Kate Tettmar (Richard Underwood)

St Albans City and District Council for a second parkrun. There was a lot to do to get it started but we had plenty of support from parkrun HQ and our local ambassador.'

From finding a suitable venue to getting the landowner's permission and designing and measuring the course, Kate said it took about a year until the first Heartwood Forest parkrun took place in the new native forest, owned and managed by the Woodland Trust. It was a big success but unfortunately had to cease running a year later after the landowner withdrew their support. The team were keen to find another venue and, after presenting their case to Sandridge Parish Council, they were given permission to use a nearby park they owned. Jersey Farm parkrun was then born in Autumn 2018 and has been going strong ever since. Kate's experience shows there can be a number of hurdles to overcome to set up a new parkrun but she said it was worth all the effort as she's so 'pleased and proud of the community we have at Jersey Farm parkrun', where she remains involved as an Event Director. Her top tips for anyone wanting to set up a parkrun are: to find a location 'that not also has a suitable course, but has a supportive landowner'; to pull together a good team – 'ideally some of whom

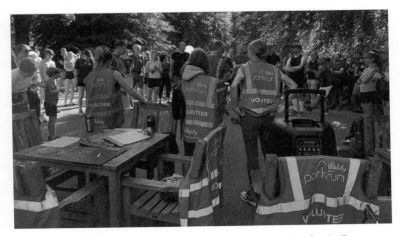

Wakehurst parkrun, whose course goes round an Elizabethan mansion (Ian Dumbrell)

will already have some experience as parkrun volunteers because starting up a parkrun is not something you can do on your own'; and keep the course design simple.

Meanwhile, Ian Dumbrell, 58, a retired financial services consultant from West Sussex, was the driving force behind Wakehurst parkrun starting in 2024, with the help of two other Event Directors. There are already a number of popular parkruns in the area but Ian always felt that Wakehurst, an estate containing beautiful gardens surrounding an Elizabethan mansion owned by the National Trust and managed by Royal Botanic Gardens, Kew, would make a fantastic parkrun venue. Thankfully both agreed, allowing the parkrun to take place before the site is open to the public, and waiving the parking fee until 11am. Ian's next task was then to devise a suitable course that would show off the amazing grounds but bypass a hill nicknamed 'the Himalayas' because it is so steep. 'I must have walked every blade of grass,' he chuckles of his course recces. 'We wanted a route that shows off the mansion, the dell, waterfalls and rhododendrons but wouldn't put people off by being too hilly.' In the end a two lap course was agreed which has had hugely positive feedback from participants and creates a great finish line atmosphere close to the cafe. Since starting in the Spring of 2024, the event has been getting more than 400 participants each week. Ian said their popularity shows that when starting a new parkrun, it is important to have a venue, course and team of volunteers who can cope with big numbers. 'I had mixed emotions seeing over 400 participants at our first event,' he recalls. 'It was a fantastic sight and proof that the venue was a popular choice. But it was also daunting for the team of volunteers, who coped admirably. It helped that many of us had already volunteered at parkruns before. I'm delighted to finally have a parkrun running at Wakehurst after thinking about it for years. It is such a wonderful location that is amazing to run around in every season.'

FURTHER READING

For more from parkrun itself, visit their official websites and social media pages:

parkrun.org.uk,
parkrun.com,
blog.parkrun.com/uk,
www.instagram.com/parkrunuk
and volunteer.parkrun.com.

Its Annual Report can be viewed here:
www.parkrun.com/about/the-organisation/annual-report

For more information on individual parkruns, each event has its own website page, for example www.parkrun.org.uk/bushy and Facebook page. The latter can be found by using the search function on Facebook or via search engines.

You can chat with fellow parkrunners on numerous unofficial Facebook groups. These include: parkrun Tourism, The parkrun discussion group, parkrun dogs, and parkrun statsgeek group

For more on various academic studies that have been carried out on parkrun, visit: https://awrcparkrunresearch.wordpress.com

For more on the Couch to 5k plan visit
www.nhs.uk/live-well/exercise/get-running-with-couch-to-5k
and download the app via app stores.

The '5k' app (the logo is a white figure running over a purple background) can be downloaded via app stores.

For more on Move Charity and 5kyourway visit movecharity.org

To view Tim Grose's full list of the UK's fastest parkruns, with thanks to him for sharing details in the Guide, visit: www.thepowerof10.info. He also discusses this and numerous other running-related topics on his YouTube channel: www.youtube.com/user/drtimgrose

THANKS

At parkrun HQ, thank you to Kirsty Woodbridge and Russ Jefferys for sharing their time to provide some information and pictures for this Guide, and Helen and her team of volunteers at Colwick parkrun for allowing me to shadow them at an event.

Thank you to the admins and various members of the unofficial Facebook groups who have contributed to this Guide.

Thank you to Dr Anne Grunseit for sharing her knowledge and research on parkrun with the Guide.

Thank you to Graham Smith for taking the cover photo and to the parkrunners pictured: Antonia, Mike and Gill Jubb, Barnaby and Megan Walker, Caroline Bailes, Errol and Jenny Maginley, Gladstone Thompson, Giles Horridge, Heather Hann, Hannah Burkhardt, Adam Yorwerth, Kate Dixon, Martha Hall, Paul Goodwin and Joe McCormick.

Finally, thank you to all the individual parkrunners who have shared their inspirational and moving stories in the guide, offered their thoughts on what they love about parkrun, and talked about their experiences as runners, walkers and volunteers. It is often said that it is not the run that makes parkrun so special but the people, and everyone who has contributed to this guide is testament to that.

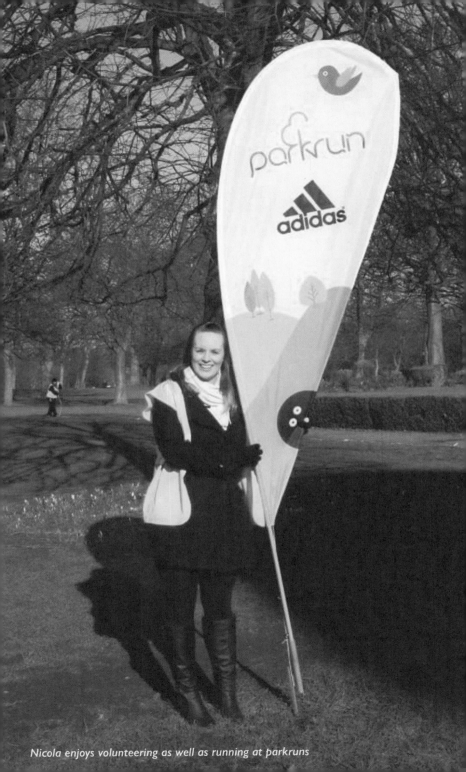

Nicola enjoys volunteering as well as running at parkruns

EPILOGUE

Someone who sums up the spirit of parkrun is Nicola Forwood, 41, a mum and Personal Trainer from Leeds. She says…

On a Saturday morning, there is no place I would rather be than at a parkrun with my daughter, Poppy, 11, by my side. To me, parkrun is much more than a free, weekly, timed 5k. It is all of the joy and passion I have for running squashed into a few hours. Without parkrun, my world would feel a lot smaller and there would be a lot less fun — and I would have missed out on meeting a lot of incredible humans.

When I attended my first parkrun 16 years ago, I could never have predicted what I was setting in motion, nor what an important role parkrun would go on to play in my life. Being a proud parkrunner has helped me through some particularly difficult times and taken me all around the world.

My parkrun journey started in November 2007 at Woodhouse Moor in Leeds (also known locally as Hyde Park). I was a student at the time and I had seen the 'Hyde Park Time Trial' advertised on a university newsletter. As it was free, I decided to check it out. Back then, it didn't resemble parkrun as we know it now. As it was a Time Trial, it was all about 'how fast can you run 5k?' I didn't enjoy this at all. I definitely didn't consider myself a runner at the time and I wasn't used to running hard. I ran all out at my maximum effort and finished in 32 minutes 30 seconds, which placed me towards the back of the field in 63rd out of 81 runners. As I struggled for breath at the finish line I wondered why I'd come. It hadn't been fun. My bed seemed a much better place to spend Saturday mornings from then on. It took me well over six months to run my second event, and that was because I wanted to challenge myself occasionally to go outside of my comfort zone running.

I was delighted when the transition from time trial to parkrun happened, and the atmosphere at events evolved along with the name. The emphasis was no longer on speed but on turning up and taking part. People of all ages and all shapes and sizes started appearing on the start line next to me: There were parents pushing running buggies, pregnant women, runners with dogs, and those running 5k for the very first time. It was clear this was no longer just a Time Trial for serious runners in short shorts (although you could still try to run as fast as you could if you wished), but a community event where everybody was welcomed with open arms. Like me, people wanted a weekly dose of fresh air, exercise and friendship.

I knew the magic of parkrun could only happen because people volunteered to help them take place, so I started doing this too. I had started running more, thanks to parkrun, and I had also joined a running club. If there was a race on a Sunday, then on Saturday I would rest and volunteer to marshal at parkrun. I loved learning people's names and cheering them on as they ran around the park. I always left feeling happy and content, with a warm fuzzy feeling in my tummy. Run or volunteer at 9am on a Saturday morning, I always had the fantastic feeling that my weekend was off to the best possible start.

My boyfriend at the time, Ben (who would later become my husband) moved up to Leeds and our house was less than a five minute walk from the start line of Woodhouse Moor parkrun. A few weeks after we had moved in together, Ben was diagnosed with a brain tumour. Being fit and healthy gave him a much better chance in his battle with cancer, so we started running together regularly. In 2008 we got engaged, and in the run up to the wedding, parkrun became my weekly ritual with my friends. In 2010, I ran parkrun on my hen do with my close friends and family. Most were non-runners and so were pretty unimpressed by having to get up early on a Saturday morning after a night out to run. But they embraced the occasion and we all ran with huge smiles on our faces. Traditionally a bride is carried over a threshold, but I ended up giving my best friend, Emma, a piggyback as her trainers had rubbed to give her a bleeding ankle. We crossed the line in fits of giggles with my fancy dress veil flapping behind me.

Ben and I got married on a beach in Sri Lanka so there was no parkrun there to build into our wedding celebrations, but as we began married life we managed to do our first bits of parkrun tourism. In 2010, this was a lot harder than it is now as events were few and far between. But to our delight, parkruns started springing up in all of the right places, so when we were visiting friends around the UK, we would parkrun. Whenever we were away for the weekend, we'd search for a local parkrun nearby. It became a theme of our lives. We found visiting different parkrun communities really rewarding. It was a great way to have mini adventures and explore little corners of the world that we might not otherwise visit.

I became pregnant with Poppy in 2012 and her very first parkrun was jiggling around in my tummy; as I was lucky enough to be able to run throughout my pregnancy. Soon after Poppy was born, Ben's condition deteriorated. He fought bravely for the next two years and took pleasure in completing parkruns as a sign of

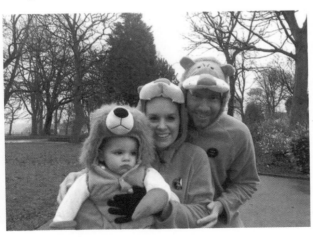

Nicola Forwood, husband Ben and daughter Poppy

strength when on chemotherapy, radiotherapy, and even the week after a craniotomy. His determination was incredibly inspiring but sadly, in 2015, aged 38, he lost his battle with cancer and left me a widowed parent to two-year-old Poppy.

During this difficult time, parkrun became my outlet. When Ben was dying, parkrun gave me something to structure my week around, and something to look forward to. It gave me a reason to get out of the hospice once a week and remember who I was, even if for only 30 minutes. It was so important for me to have this Saturday morning access to my running community at a time when I felt very alone, scared, and isolated. It was a place to laugh, and a place to cry. A place to be just a face in a crowd, and a place to be held by my local community – parkrun was whatever I needed it to be. Everyone was so supportive, and it was a huge comfort to be surrounded by a community that loved Ben so very much. The week after he died, we held a celebration of his life at Woodhouse Moor parkrun. Hundreds of runners pinned pictures of Ben to their chest and Poppy completed her first ever full parkrun, scanning her Daddy's barcode at the finish line for one final time. There were many tears of sadness, but also tears of joy as we ran and remembered happy memories of a very special man.

After Ben's death, I had posthumous IVF to have a sibling for Poppy. I was over the moon when the procedure worked and I got pregnant. The feeling didn't last long, I came crashing down to earth and was absolutely devastated when I lost the baby at 16 weeks. Feeling distraught, I knew I needed to get away, but I still needed to feel connected to my life with Ben. Once again parkrun was my salvation. I took Poppy on a parkrun tour 'Down Under'. We started by running two parkruns in New Zealand. At one on the North Island – Cornwall Park parkrun – we felt very much like we were at home, because the Run Director, Jeff, was a Yorkshireman I knew well from Leeds! Proof it is a small parkrun world! Our run on the South Island at Blenheim parkrun was somewhat different. We were standing on the start line alone and with 10 minutes to go I was panicking thinking 'where is everyone?'. Then all of a sudden a few people arrived, popped up a finish funnel and we were good to go! What a relief! Poppy and I finished last in positions 33 and 34 on that occasion as these were the days before compulsory Tail Walkers.

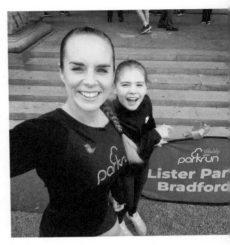

Nicola and Poppy have visited numerous parkruns

We then ran four parkruns in Australia. St Peters parkrun in Sydney was the first and was a pretty hilly course. The team had written the best motivational messages on the floor in chalk such as 'I KNOW I CAN' near the start, 'NEARLY THERE' towards the top of a hill, and 'YOU DID IT, GREAT JOB' before the finish. We needed the encouragement, as there was a heatwave at the time, and despite it being early in the morning it was already 26 degrees when we started running.

The following Saturday we headed to Melbourne to stay with friends and together took our kids to Chelsea Bicenten-

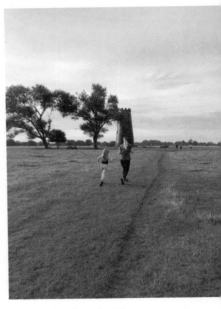

nial parkrun, followed by an afternoon on the beach. It's a pretty cool parkrun life down under! Cairns parkrun in Queensland was next and it was unreal. Looking out over the ocean to incredible mountains, palm trees, giant shell sculptures, stunning flowers, and even signs to warn of the dangers of crocodiles! It started at 7am but it was sweltering. Luckily there was a kids' splash park outside the cafe so Poppy could cool off. Noosa parkrun, also in Queensland, was our final parkrun in Australia. I think it was my favourite of the trip as I was fascinated by the Scribbly Gum trees we ran past, plus a kind lady gave Poppy a dog on a lead to run with. Poppy was over the moon with her new found responsibility as a temporary dog owner and squealed with delight the entire run. On the way back from our antipodean adventure, Poppy ran her 10th parkrun, age four, at a very hot and humid East Coast Park parkrun in Singapore. It was beautiful. Lined with palm trees it tracked the coast on an out-and-back course with footprints painted on the tarmac that Poppy just loved following. The trip had been a life-affirming adventure and the reset I so badly needed. By travelling to different parkruns in different countries, I was able to show my daughter that people are kind, loving, and warm; that integrating into different communities is a blessing; and the world is our oyster.

Back home, I carried on parkrunning across the UK. For me, it became a comforting constant. Something that I could rely on, that I could look forward to and build my week around. I've been to numerous beautiful parkrun venues. I love parkruns at National Trust properties and one of my absolute favourites is Fountains Abbey parkrun in Yorkshire. This runs around the ruined Abbey itself but also around Studley Royal Water Garden. The grounds are incredible at this beautiful UNESCO World Heritage site and it feels a real privilege to be able to parkrun here.

For my 40th birthday in 2023, Poppy and I went on another big parkrun adventure. I sold my car, bought a camper van, and we travelled around the coast of Ireland for three months, hopping from parkrun community to parkrun community, meeting countless incredible people along the way. It was during this trip that I found my favourite ever parkrun – Bere Island in County Cork. It is breathtakingly beautiful, surrounded by the sea with views of stunning mountains, and there is a very special island vibe. You need to get a ferry, and a minibus (usually travelling in convoy depending on the number of visiting parkrunners) to the start line which makes it an even more exciting parkrun experience! It will always have a special place in my heart.

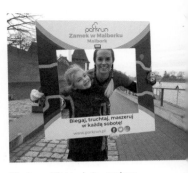

Nicola and Poppy being parkrun tourists

I have now run more than 650 parkruns at over 200 different venues. Over the years parkrun milestones to me have come to represent resilience, determination, and a commitment to my passion. I wear my 500 club T-shirt with pride. It will take me another seven years to reach my next milestone of 1,000 and I'm looking forward to seeing where these seven years will take me. I am so proud that Poppy has grown up being part of it all – parkrun has shown her that when people come together to create a community over a shared passion, then incredible things can happen. We have run in 12 different countries together and we now have a huge network of people I am proud to call our parkrun family. She has racked up some valuable life experience and seen so much of the world with more than 200 parkruns to her name at over 125 different locations.

parkrun is a way for us to have an adventure every Saturday morning – some big and some small – but all incredibly fulfilling and life-affirming. I can't imagine my life without it. Long may our parkrunning adventures continue.

Nicola shares her parkrun travels on her YouTube channel @NicolaRuns

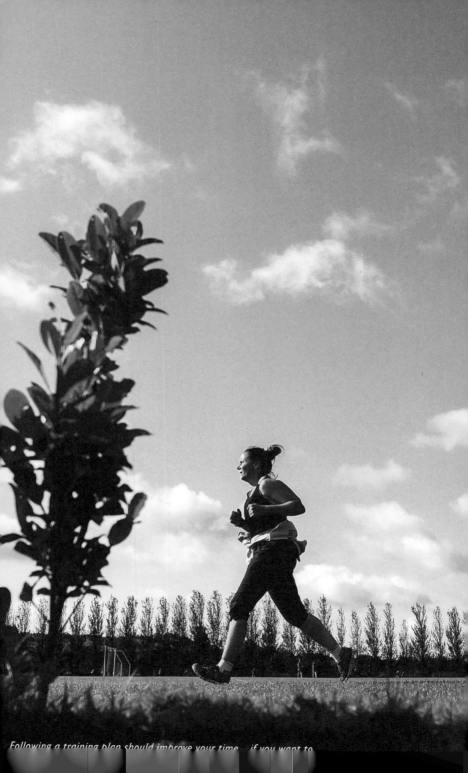

Following a training plan should improve your time — if you want to

TRAINING PLANS

SUB 30: THIS PLAN CAN BE FOLLOWED AFTER COMPLETING THE COUCH TO 5K PLAN.

> ➤ If you miss a week, repeat the week where you left off before progressing.
> ➤ You can parkrun every week following this plan (if you want to) but save hard efforts for weeks 4 and 8 to maximise your chance to run well, aiming for week 8's parkrun to be faster than week 4's

	MON	TUES**	WED	THURS	FRI	SAT	SUN
1	*Strength and conditioning exercises	5min, 4min, 3min, 2min, 1min hard efforts, with 90 seconds walk/slow jog in between each	Rest	30 minutes easy***	Strength and conditioning exercises	Easy parkrun or solo easy 5k run	Rest
2	Strength and conditioning exercises	1min hard, 1 min easy x 10	Rest	30 minutes easy***	Strength and conditioning exercises	Easy parkrun or solo easy 5k run	Rest
3		4 x 2 min uphill, jog back down, 4 x 30 sec uphill, jog back down	Rest	35 minutes easy***	Strength and conditioning exercises	Easy parkrun or solo easy 5k run	Rest
4	Strength and conditioning exercises	4 x 1k hard, 2 min walk/slow jog in between	Rest	35 minutes easy, + 4 x 15 second strides****	Rest	Hard effort parkrun*****	Rest
5	Strength and conditioning exercises	2 min, 4 min, 6 min, 4 min, 2 min hard, 2 min walk/slow jog in between	Rest	40 minutes easy***	Strength and conditioning exercises	Easy parkrun or solo easy 5k run	Rest
6	Strength and conditioning exercises	3 x 1 mile hard, 2 min walk/slow jog in between	Rest	45 minutes easy***	Strength and conditioning exercises	Easy parkrun or solo easy 5k run	Rest
7	Strength and conditioning exercises	4 x 2 min uphill, jog back down, 4 x 30 sec uphill, jog back down	Rest	45 minutes easy***	Strength and conditioning exercises	Easy parkrun or solo easy 5k run	Rest
8	Strength and conditioning exercises	8 x 2 min hard, 1 min walk/slow jog in between	Rest	30 minutes easy + 4 x 15 second strides ****	Rest	Hard effort parkrun*****	Rest

* Strength and conditioning exercises: See if you can join in a local Pilates/gym class or online class for this. Or do each of these exercises for 2 x 30 seconds with 30 seconds break in between: Squats, lunges, glute bridges, sit ups, planks, calf raises, crab walks, dead bug, press ups. Search online for exercise demonstrations. Progress to using weights and/or resistance band as you get stronger.

** All Tues sessions should be sandwiched between a 10 minute slow warm up jog, and 10 minute cool down jog.

*** Easy pace is when your heart rate isn't too high and you can comfortably hold a conversation while running.

**** Strides means running fast, almost a sprint focusing on good running form.

***** Hard effort is pushing yourself to run faster, heart rate high, only able to talk in short bursts because breathing is heavy eg just enough breath to say 'thanks marshal!' when you pass one.

SUB 25: THIS PLAN CAN BE FOLLOWED BY RUNNERS WHO HAVE ALREADY RUN A SUB 30MIN 5K

- If you miss a week, repeat the week where you left off before progressing.
- You can parkrun every week following this plan (if you want to) by swapping the Saturday sessions to Thursday in weeks 1-3 and 5-7, and then keeping the parkrun at an easy pace on those weeks.
- If you're only used to/only have time for running four times a week, make Wednesday a rest day.

WEEK		MON	TUES**	WED	THURS	FRI	SAT	SUN
	1	*Strength and conditioning exercises	5min, 4min, 3min, 2min, 1min hard efforts with 90 seconds walk/slow jog in between each	Rest or 30 min easy***	30 minutes easy plus Strength and conditioning exercises	Rest	Continuous 50 min progression run****: 10 min easy warm up 10 min marathon pace 10 min half marathon pace 10 min 10k pace 10 min easy cool down	70 min easy
	2	Strength and conditioning exercises	1min hard, 1 min easy x 12	Rest or 30 min easy***	35 minutes easy plus Strength and conditioning exercises	Rest	Continuous fartlek 10 min easy warm up 3 mins 10k pace, 3 mins a minute slower than that pace x 4 10 mins easy cool down	70 min easy
	3	Strength and conditioning exercises	5 x 2 min uphill, jog back down, 5 x 30 sec uphill, jog back down	Rest or 30 min easy***	40 minutes easy plus Strength and conditioning exercises	Rest	10 min warm up 3 x 10 minute reps with 2 min walk/slow jog in between 10 min cool down	75 min easy
	4	Strength and conditioning exercises	5 x 1k hard, 2 min walk/slow jog in between	Rest or 30 min easy***	30 minutes easy plus 4 x 15 second strides*****	Rest	Hard effort parkrun******	60 min easy
	5	Strength and conditioning exercises	2 min, 4 min, 6 min, 4 min, 2 min hard, 2 min walk/slow jog in between	Rest or 30 min easy***	40 minutes easy plus Strength and conditioning exercises	Rest	Continuous 50 min progression run****: 10 min easy warm up 10 min marathon pace 10 min half marathon pace 10 min 10k pace 10 min easy cool down	75 min easy
	6	Strength and conditioning exercises	4 x 1 mile, 2 min walk/slow jog in between	Rest or 30 min easy***	40 minutes easy plus Strength and conditioning exercises	Rest	Continuous fartlek 10 min easy warm up 3 mins 10k pace, 3 mins a minute slower than that pace x 4 10 mins easy cool down	80 min easy
	7	Strength and conditioning exercises	5 x 2 min uphill, jog back down, 5 x 30 sec uphill, jog back down	Rest or 30 min easy***	40 minutes easy plus Strength and conditioning exercises	Rest	10 min warm up 5 x 5 minute reps with 2 min walk/slow jog in between 10 min cool down	80 min easy
	8	Strength and conditioning exercises	8 x 2 min, 1 min walk/slow jog in between	Rest or 30 min easy***	30 minutes easy + 4 x 15 second strides*****	Rest	Hard effort parkrun******	60 min easy

* Strength and conditioning exercises: See if you can join in a local Pilates/gym class or online class for this. Or do each of these exercises for 2 x 30 seconds with 30 seconds break in between: Squats, lunges, glute bridges, sit ups, planks, calf raises, crab walks, dead bug, press ups. Search online for exercise demonstrations. Progress to using weights and/or resistance band as you get stronger.

** All Tues sessions should be sandwiched between a 10 minute slow warm up jog, and 10 minute cool down jog.

*** Easy pace is when your heart rate isn't too high and you can comfortably hold a conversation while running.

**** Search for an online pace calculator to work these out using a recent PB time if you're not sure what yours are for each distance.

***** Strides means running fast, almost a sprint focusing on good running form.

****** Hard effort is pushing yourself to run faster, heart rate high, only able to talk in short bursts because breathing is heavy eg just enough breath to say 'thanks marshal!' when you pass one.

SUB 20: THIS PLAN CAN BE FOLLOWED BY RUNNERS WHO HAVE ALREADY RUN A SUB 25MIN 5K

> ➤ If you miss a week, repeat the week where you left off before progressing.
> ➤ You can parkrun every week following this plan (if you want to) by swapping the Saturday sessions in weeks 1-3 and weeks 5-7 to Thursday, and adding an easy 10 min warm up and 10 min cool down around doing an easy parkrun on those weeks

WEEK	MON	TUES**	WED	THURS	FRI	SAT	SUN
1	*Strength and conditioning exercises	6min, 5min, 4min, 3min, 2min, 1min hard efforts with 90 seconds walk/slow jog in between each	30 min easy***	45 minutes easy plus Strength and conditioning exercises	Rest	Continuous 65 min progression run****: 10 min easy warm up 15 min marathon pace 15 min half marathon pace 15 min 10k pace 10 min easy cool down	80 mins easy
2	Strength and conditioning exercises	1min hard, 1 min easy x 15	30 min easy***	45 minutes easy plus Strength and conditioning exercises	Rest	Continuous fartlek 10 min easy warm up 3 mins 10k pace, 3 mins a minute slower than that pace x 5 10 mins easy cool down	80 mins easy
3	Strength and conditioning exercises	5 x 2 min uphill, jog back down, 5 x 30 sec uphill, jog back down	30 min easy***	50 minutes easy plus Strength and conditioning exercises	Rest	10 min warm up 3 x 10 minute reps with 2 min walk/slow jog in between 10 min cool down	80 mins easy
4	Strength and conditioning exercises	6 x 1k hard, 2 min walk/slow jog in between	30 min easy	30 minutes easy plus 4 x 15 second strides*****	Rest	Hard effort parkrun******	60 mins easy
5	Strength and conditioning exercises	2 min, 4 min, 6 min, 4 min, 2 min hard, 2 min walk/slow jog in between	30 min easy***	60 minutes easy plus Strength and conditioning exercises	Rest	Continuous 65 min progression run****: 10 min easy warm up 15 min marathon pace 15 min half marathon pace 15 min 10k pace 10 min easy cool down	90 mins easy
6	Strength and conditioning exercises	5 x 1 mile, 2 min walk/slow jog in between	30 min easy***	60 minutes easy plus Strength and conditioning exercises	Rest	Continuous fartlek 10 min easy warm up 3 mins 10k pace, 3 mins a minute slower than that pace x 5 10 mins easy cool down	90 mins easy
7	Strength and conditioning exercises	6 x 2 min uphill, jog back down, 6 x 30 sec uphill, jog back down	30 min easy***	60 minutes easy plus Strength and conditioning exercises	Rest	10 min warm up 6 x 5 minute reps with 2 min walk/slow jog in between 10 min cool down	90 mins easy
8	Strength and conditioning exercises	8 x 2 min, 1 min walk/slow jog in between	30 min easy***	30 minutes easy + 4 x 15 second strides*****	Rest	Hard effort parkrun******	60 mins easy

* Strength and conditioning exercises: See if you can join in a local Pilates/gym class or online class for this. Or do each of these exercises for 2 x 30 seconds with 30 seconds break in between: Squats, lunges, glute bridges, sit ups, planks, calf raises, crab walks, dead bug, press ups. Search online for exercise demonstrations. Progress to using weights and/or resistance band as you get stronger.
** All Tues sessions should be sandwiched between a 10 minute slow warm up jog, and 10 minute cool down jog.
*** Easy pace is when your heart rate isn't too high and you can comfortably hold a conversation while running.
**** Search for an online pace calculator to work these out using a recent PB time if you're not sure what yours are for each distance.
***** Strides means running fast, almost a sprint focusing on good running form.
****** Hard effort is pushing yourself to run faster, heart rate high, only able to talk in short bursts because breathing is heavy eg just enough breath to say 'thanks marshal!' when you pass one.

More from Canbury Press

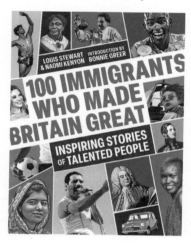

100 Immigrants Who Made Britain Great
Inspiring Stories of Talented People
Louis Stewart, Naomi Kenyon,
ISBN: 9781914487460

A beautifully illustrated book celebrating the achievements
of 100 inspirational characters who made a new life
in Britain. From T. S. Eliot to Malala, Mo Farah to Jimi
Hendrix, each has a biography and colour illustration.

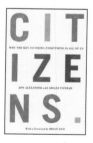

Citizens
Jon Alexander
ISBN: 9781912454884

How, together, we can solve
big problems.
FT: 'An underground hit'